EMBERS OF CONFIDENCE

HOW I TRAINED THREE FEMALE SMOKEJUMPERS

BY FRITZ NUGENT

MS, MA, CSCS, CCFT, USAW, SFG1

WHAT PEOPLE ARE SAYING

"An extremely smart and powerful reflection of what it means to be a coach. I'm not only honored to be mentioned in this book, but it was so thought-provoking and engaging that I felt as if I was hovering over Fritz's life as an athlete, coach, husband, and father. It shows the day-to-day struggles and sacrifices of his personal journey which exemplifies what it takes to be awarded the title "Coach." His step-by-step analysis and technical diaries are not only a glimpse of what it takes to be successful, but a learning tool for all current and aspiring coaches. This book is an intelligent example of how to unlock your athlete's full potential. Congrats Fritz on a job well done."

– Tonja Buford-Bailey, three-time track and field Olympian

"On the surface, this book is a fascinating account of three determined, capable, bad ass women and their aspirations to become smokejumpers. Fritz did a phenomenal job of describing their training journey in a way that both experts and laymen would enjoy. Each woman was different, but the common theme of confidence, courage, and a dash of crazy was both inspirational and monumentally impressive.

As a coach myself, I identified most with the way he described his own process with such openness and vulnerability. We often read accounts of coaches and mentors who look back on their experiences with great confidence in their plans. The truth is, even the most accomplished coaches and trainers still work with a degree of uncertainty. No two athletes respond the same way to training stimuli, and we can never predict how life outside of training affects results. In Fritz's case, he wasn't even a firefighter, much less a smokejumper. While he is an accomplished sport coach, this endeavor would be akin to understanding how to sail a boat but not having any idea of the ocean conditions that lay ahead. It's here, along with thoughtful and poignant personal anecdotes smartly interwoven with technical narrative, that this book really shines.

Whether you're an aspiring smokejumper, a coach, or just someone who enjoys well told true stories about inspirational efforts, you'll thoroughly enjoy this book. These tales deserve to be told, and I hope Fritz continues to document the success of both he and his athletes."

– Mike Erb, Assistant Track & Field Coach, Indiana University

EMBERS OF CONFIDENCE

HOW I TRAINED THREE FEMALE SMOKEJUMPERS

BY FRITZ NUGENT

MS, MA, CSCS, CCFT, USAW, SFG1

FNP

DEDICATION

This book is dedicated to my daughter, Fiona.

ACKNOWLEDGEMENTS

I put off finishing this section to the very end because the list of people who have helped me bring this book to life keeps growing. First off, Heidi. She got me into all this. My deepest gratitude goes out to her. Sierra comes next, of course. And just like the chapters in the book, next, I am grateful for Cameron. For a while there, Cam didn't want her story published. She said even if I wrote this book with a fake name for her, she is the only female smokejumping for Alaska; it wouldn't take a genius to figure out who she is. After she realized this book could increase interest in wildland fire, and hopefully inspire more females to join, she agreed that her story (through my eyes, of course) is worthy of telling. Thank you, Heidi, Sierra, and Cameron. I could not have written this book without you.

Next comes Mike and Tonja. I learned so much about coaching and life from each of you. Much of my coaching success can be attributed to the lessons I learned while working with you both.

Pavel. I've been reading your books for over twenty years. A large chunk of my foundational strength and conditioning knowledge comes from your texts. Thank you for leading the way. You also inspired me to write this book by pulling me on stage at the Programming Improv seminar, and you made my year by following up with me. Because of you, I learned that what the women and I had accomplished was impressive and worthy of writing about.

This book would have been a textbook if it wasn't for my developmental editors, Nadia Geagea Pupa and Lindsay Denney. Nadia read through my first draft and suggested I start over and tell my story, and months later after I transformed my textbook into a story, Lindsay helped me dial in the emotional details. Thank you to Maris Williams, my copyeditor. Last, but certainly not least, Rachelle Funk, my proofreader. She was the last line of defense before publication and I'm very grateful that Nadia connected us. Rachelle put the finishing editorial touches on the book to make it shine.

A special thank you goes out to my wife for allowing me to write about her liberally in this book. As of one-month pre-publication, Jess has read none of this. Hopefully, she doesn't hate it. Her close friends will get a kick out of her character, and those who don't know her well might be very confused.

Thank you, young Travis, for making sure I kept up with my writing and for your read-through from a coach's eye. Thank you, Mom and Dad, for checking on me each week about this book (and for everything else that one can thank their parents for). You held me accountable, ensuring this book was eventually completed.

For many amazing reasons, thank you to my daughter for being born. Because of you, I got to take time off work, and I used some of that time to finish this book.

And lastly, thank you to YOU, the reader. I hope you find this book funny, interesting, and inspiring. Through your support, I was able to become an author, something that I have wanted to be for my entire life.

MESSAGE FROM THE AUTHOR

At first glance, the title of this book might strike you, the reader, as ill-fitting or, perhaps, a bit misleading. Embers are what remain when a fire dies, right? Wouldn't "Ignition of Confidence" or "Blazing Confidence" make more sense as titles? Before delving into the book, those options may seem appropriate. However, I believe they fail to capture the essence of this story.

Let's journey back thousands of years and explore a different understanding of embers and how they were used. Our ancestors knew the secret of a remarkable mushroom-based felt called amadou. When hollowed out, it possessed unique properties allowing the transportation and reutilization of embers from the previous evening's fire. For them, transporting and reigniting embers represented opportunities for intercontinental migration, starting anew, and chasing the horizon.

The people within these pages, including myself, experienced unique character arcs where our individual flames ran out of fuel, leaving only smoldering embers. We each began our journeys with limited confidence, wondering what was possible for ourselves. But through grit and perseverance, we reignited those embers into blazing fires of success, happiness, and meaning.

As you read, I hope this book serves as tinder to ignite the embers within yourself. To paraphrase a respected colleague, "See the potential for a great life and have the courage to pursue it." Godspeed.

CONTENTS

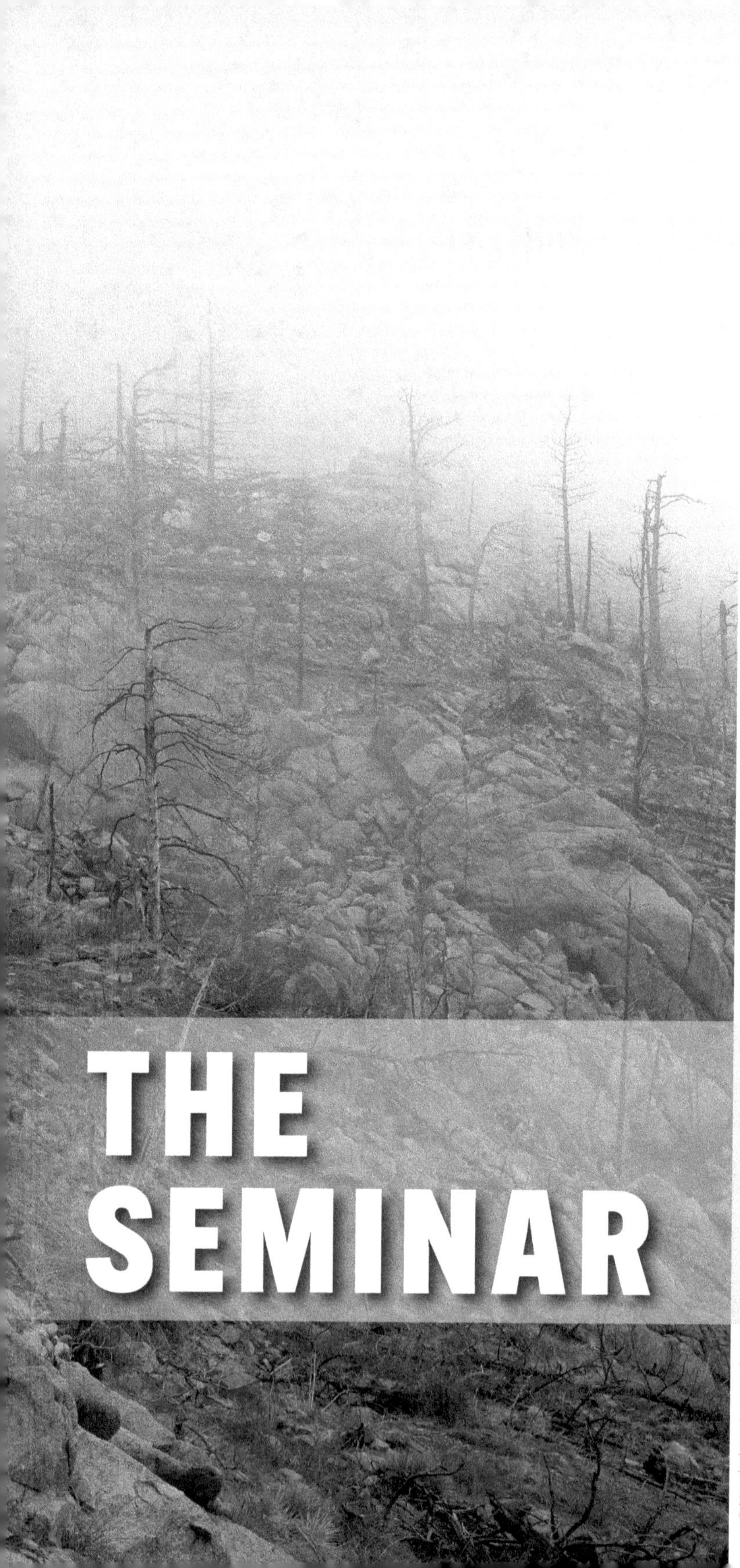

1 THE SEMINAR

I HAD A PIT IN MY GUT. Aching. I knew that something was going to happen, but I didn't know what. I felt that I had to act, but I was terrified to learn the consequences of submitting my athlete's data to Pavel Tsatsouline and his team. Pavel is one of the top strength and conditioning professionals on the planet. Pavel "The Evil Russian": the man who first popularized kettlebells in the United States in the early 2000s, who has written dozens of top-selling fitness books, who runs a strength and conditioning company called StrongFirst, and travels all over the world teaching his methods to coaches like myself in seminars like the one I was currently involved in.

Pavel made his name by coaching Russian Special Forces athletes and deciphering the findings and teachings of famous Russian sport scientists into simple and effective strength training principles and programs for Americans to follow and learn from. Russian sport scientists are famous in the strength and conditioning and Olympic sport communities for discovering many of the world's exercise science breakthroughs between 1950 and 1990. Many of the principles that coaches, trainers, and health practitioners rely upon today to coach and train their athletes were first tested, tweaked, and perfected during this explosive and fruitful phase of Soviet sport science exploration.

> Plyometrics, initially named, "shock method" or "shock training", was first explored by Russian sport scientist Yuri Verkhoshansky in Russia in 1959 and published in the *Bulletin of the Central Research Institute of Physical Culture*. The method originally prioritized the depth jump. Today, there are endless variations of plyometric training tasks.

Perhaps the greatest discovery to arise from this magnificent era was plyometrics, which has since been proven the most potent and effective methodology for preparing explosive athletes for competition on the world stage, especially in the realm of track and field where the capacities of speed and power are maximally tested through worldwide competition. The limiting factor for decades was that many of the sport science texts from this time and the training secrets contained within them were only available in the Russian language. Pavel grew up in Russia and was fortunate to study these texts and brought the Soviet strength, power, and endurance training methodology to the West, successfully leveraging his exclusivity to this unique knowledge as a marketing tactic. It worked.

Pavel has done quite well for himself, and many others have improved their lives and conquered incredible physical feats using his translated, tested, and packaged methodologies. I am most impressed by his ability to simplify the scientific complexities for everyday folks, empowering people to take back or improve their health.

I traveled from San Diego to Denver for a short weekend to learn and grow no matter how painful the experience might be. I submitted my athlete's data for critique. I genuinely wanted to learn how I could become a more effective coach. I was also eager about what I might learn. What if I discovered that my athletes were successful despite my coaching and not because of it? That was a real possibility, and I was about to find out.

On the second day of a seminar about creating training programs for athletes, I was exhausted and fighting a cold from travel and lack of sleep. The alcohol from the night before didn't help. As is customary at these events, the evening before, completing the first day of the seminar, everyone went out for a big group dinner to socialize and talk about life outside of strength training. Even Pavel joined in the fun, sitting at the next table surrounded by a gaggle of coaches from all over the world, each eager to soak up his attention and wisdom.

About thirty of us filled the private room at the restaurant. After a mentally draining first day of the seminar, I was starving and demolished a rib eye steak covered in brown sugar butter and put back a few glasses of High West Double Rye on the rocks while I learned that the coach sitting across the table from me had recently trained for and lifted the Dinnie Stones, a pair of famous Scottish stones weighing over 700 pounds. The list of people who have lifted these stones a is short one. He wasn't a large guy, either. I found it respectable that he didn't bring any of this up himself. Others asked him about his feat, and he humbly answered their questions. As I sat in the back room of this upscale Italian restaurant in a random South Denver neighborhood, I marveled at the amount of world-class coaching talent sitting in this single room. I became overwhelmed, surrounded by Pavel's top dogs from around the world. Later that night, I heard that this group was his top echelon of coaches, and the day before this seminar, they had had a strategic in-person meeting for the first time since before the pandemic. The more I listened, the less I said as the alcohol went down for us all.

I sat on a metal folding chair as Pavel taught on day two. The day before, Pavel had laid the contextual groundwork by discussing the strength principles upon which he bases all the decisions that go into creating his training programs. Today was to illustrate the real-time application of that knowledge with case studies of other coaches' athletes submitted about a month before.

It was a silent room despite the size of the place. Through his microphone, only Pavel audibly existed. I had been reading his books for more than twenty years. In high school, I was a lanky kid. A bean pole. At 6'3" and 165 pounds, my mom knew that I wanted to put on some muscle mass to support my transition to college football the following year, so she bought me one of his books. This was 2000, before you could Google training programs producing tons of hits from coaches all over the world. She purchased *Power to the People*. Not specifically a mass-building book (it was strength-oriented and focused on only two lifts—the deadlift and the single arm barbell press), it nevertheless initiated my interest in Pavel, and I have been following him in awe ever since. Throughout my coaching career, I have attended a few StrongFirst certifications and seminars, but I had yet to meet the man in person. A few months before, I saw that he was going to be at this very event, and that solidified my decision to give up a weekend and travel to Denver. I wanted to meet him and to learn how I could become a better programmer and coach.

I now had the sniffles, and the post-nasal drip was running down into my throat, and it itched, and all I wanted to do was clear it out with an "unh huh ha" sound and cough it up. It would feel so good to do that. But I held it in, for hours, uncomfortable in the front row while partially blocking the view of those behind me. I barely kept myself together, waiting over a day and a half for Pavel to mention my athlete. I couldn't wait a moment longer to hear him discuss his solutions to her situation. This seminar, titled "Programming Improv," featured athlete case studies submitted by attendees. A month before, I had submitted data for one of my own athletes, a female smoke-jumper candidate. How would he solve the problems that I had encountered? Would he have her do more volume? Less? A different progression entirely? How would he vary the exercise selection? When would he add in weighted calisthenics, and how would he layer in the volume? There was no guarantee that he would discuss her at all. I had a feeling that he would, though. How could he pass on a chance to talk about how he'd train something as rare as a female smokejumper?!

A smokejumper is an elite wildland firefighter. Smokejumpers are often the first line of defense against forest fires. They fly to the spot of the blaze and parachute in with enough supplies for up to three self-sufficient days. Fire trucks and thousands of gallons of water are unavailable in the middle of nowhere, so these rugged mountain athletes suppress the fire's spread using hand tools to create a fire "break" by felling trees and scraping brush away, cutting off the fire's fuel supply. Once the job is done, they hike out to a fire road, sometimes a full day hike or further, are picked up in vehicles, and speed away.

When I submitted my case study, I genuinely wanted to learn how to improve my approach with training these athletes. I had been successful, but it always felt serendipitous, like a happy accident. Perhaps I had simply been blessed with amazing athletes. That's one of the interesting things that I do for my profession—I create niche training programs. In the past, I have created training programs for a broad range of sports and athletes, from technical drills for cyclocross (a mixture of hiking and mountain biking) to obstacle course racing (Spartans, and the like). For a few years, I was the strength and conditioning coach for California's strongest lightweight female strong woman, and she was crowned champion two years in a row. One of the rarest groups I train are female wildland firefighters, specifically smokejumpers. I program for male wildland firefighters as well, but once you help a female conquer a big goal, she tells other females, word spreads, and the serious ones find me.

Coaching athletes through the wildland fire physical preparation process is extremely challenging and immensely rewarding. When a smokejumper is hired, there is a good chance they are already a seasoned wildland firefighting veteran with at least five years of experience. To complete the smokejumper hiring process, the contracts of new hires are upheld when candidates graduate from a maximally taxing 5–6-week smokejumper crash course called rookie training, containing insane volumes of running, rucking, calisthenics, and parachuting technique and cadence. The rookies are mostly men, ranging from mid-twenties to mid-thirties, 150-200 pounds, and fit as hell.

During rookie training each year, every class has "wash-outs": those that fail to meet the physical requirements, others that cannot mentally handle the pressure, and some that become injured. The process is dangerous. I have spoken with rookies who washed out and headed straight to the hospital for a few days after experiencing rhabdomyolysis or acute bronchitis. Rookie training is not to be taken lightly, no matter how physically able and mentally strong someone thinks they are. After a failed dose of rookie training, sometimes the washouts take a year or more to physically recover from the experience before going back. Some never attempt it again.

And that's just the initial training process. The job itself is physically grueling. Navy Seal, Army Ranger, author, Guinness World Record holder, and general badass, David Goggins, tested himself as a smokejumper simply because he found the work to be some of the most difficult that he could find anywhere in the world.

I enjoy the challenge of preparing any smokejumper, but I especially relish the opportunity to prepare women for this traditionally male-dominated arena. Women are notable (or significant) underdogs going into the physically demanding smokejumper rookie training. In 2021, out of about 200 Bureau of Land Management (BLM) smokejumpers in the United States, three were female. That's one point five percent. The United States Forest Service (USFS) also has smokejumper bases: at the Missoula smokejumper base in Montana, there are 6-7 females; Redmond has 2 women; and West Yellowstone has a couple as well. That brings the total in the United States to about 15 women out of 400, comprising less than four percent of the workforce. Until the beginning of 2023, the women have been held to the same physical standards as the men. If they can hack it, they earn their place as a smokejumper. If they can't hold their own, they wash out, just like the men who aren't up to the standard. The physical demands of the job are extreme, and rookie training weeds out those who would be a danger to themselves or others out in the middle of the American backcountry fighting forest fires.

"Our next case study is about a female smokejumper..." Pavel's words sent a surge of adrenaline through my body, culminating with my palms sweating and my heart thumping against my ribcage. My body was entering fight or flight. My athlete!! He's talking about my athlete!!! I knew this was my time. What if he called on me to answer a question about her? What would I say? Where would I start? There is so much.

Then something unexpected occurred. His brow furrowed, indicating confusion. He stated that this particular female athlete's goals seemed unrealistic given the 6-month time constraint. He then turned to his left and asked someone in the crowd for their opinion. "Mike, you work with Navy Seals. Do these numbers seem realistic given her starting point and the limited time to prepare her?" Mike responded by saying no, it didn't seem possible given the demands and the time constraint and the fact that even his male Navy Seal candidates would have trouble hitting her goal numbers.

My jaw dropped. I literally could not believe what had just happened. My coaching idol, the man whose books I had been soaking up for twenty years stood before me and thought that what I had done was improbable. I was giddy with excitement! I must tell him that it's not only possible, that it had been done. I had been a part of it! As I sat thinking these rapid-fire thoughts in a fraction of a second, overcome with emotion, I then realized the moment was fading. I might miss an opportunity to make an impression on this man. It was now or never. I had to act, but I was momentarily frozen. My heart was jumping out of my chest. A bead of sweat formed on my temple and ran down the side of my face, so I used my shoulder to wipe it away. I knew that I had to say something. I felt simultaneously terrified and compelled. It would be easiest to say nothing, to let Pavel and his crew of excellent coaches hash out how to handle my athlete's training program. After all, they are the professionals with all the books and athletes and experience. Who was I to anyone in that room? Just some guy. And if I spoke, they would all immediately sense my imposter syndrome. How could they not? I began to feel like I was leaving my body, slipping into the passenger seat of my own life, watching myself do nothing when I knew that I should act. This had happened before in other stressful situations. Public speaking. Job interviews. My consciousness began to float up towards the ceiling to watch the show, safely tucked away from the stress of the moment. *NOOOO!* A primal voice from deep within my soul screamed out, and, as if animated on its own, my hand steadily rose into the air.

Pavel turned towards me, along with everyone else in the place. I could feel their eyes, the tension immense. I tasted battery acid on my tongue. Was this career suicide? Confusion rippled through the attendees. Before now, none of the other case studies seemed impossible. Adding stress, I knew this seminar was being broadcast live to viewers all over the world. He called on me. "We have a question over here." With all the power that I could summon, I said to him and the group, "This is my case study. I have done this with three females." I felt the air leave the room. The silence was deafening and seemed to last an eternity. Everyone froze, wondering what would come next.

For only an instant, I felt the weight of a heavy kettlebell lift off my chest. I had said my piece, and now I could sit back and learn. However, my participation in this experience was not over. At the sound of Pavel's voice, I was startled back into the stress of the moment.

Pavel read the name tag on my chest and said, "Francis, why don't you come up and teach us how you did it." It wasn't a question. I was shocked and elated. My nerves surged once more. I felt my armpits well with perspiration. My body temperature seemed to shoot up a few degrees. I shook my head and smiled, pressed my hands into my thighs to stand up, and headed towards Pavel. Someone handed me a lapel microphone, and I pinned it to my shirt at the neckline. There I was, invited up onto the seminar stage by my coaching idol. I then proceeded to teach everyone at the seminar—and those watching around the world—how I managed to prepare three females for overcoming the rigors of smokejumper rookie training.

2

HEIDI

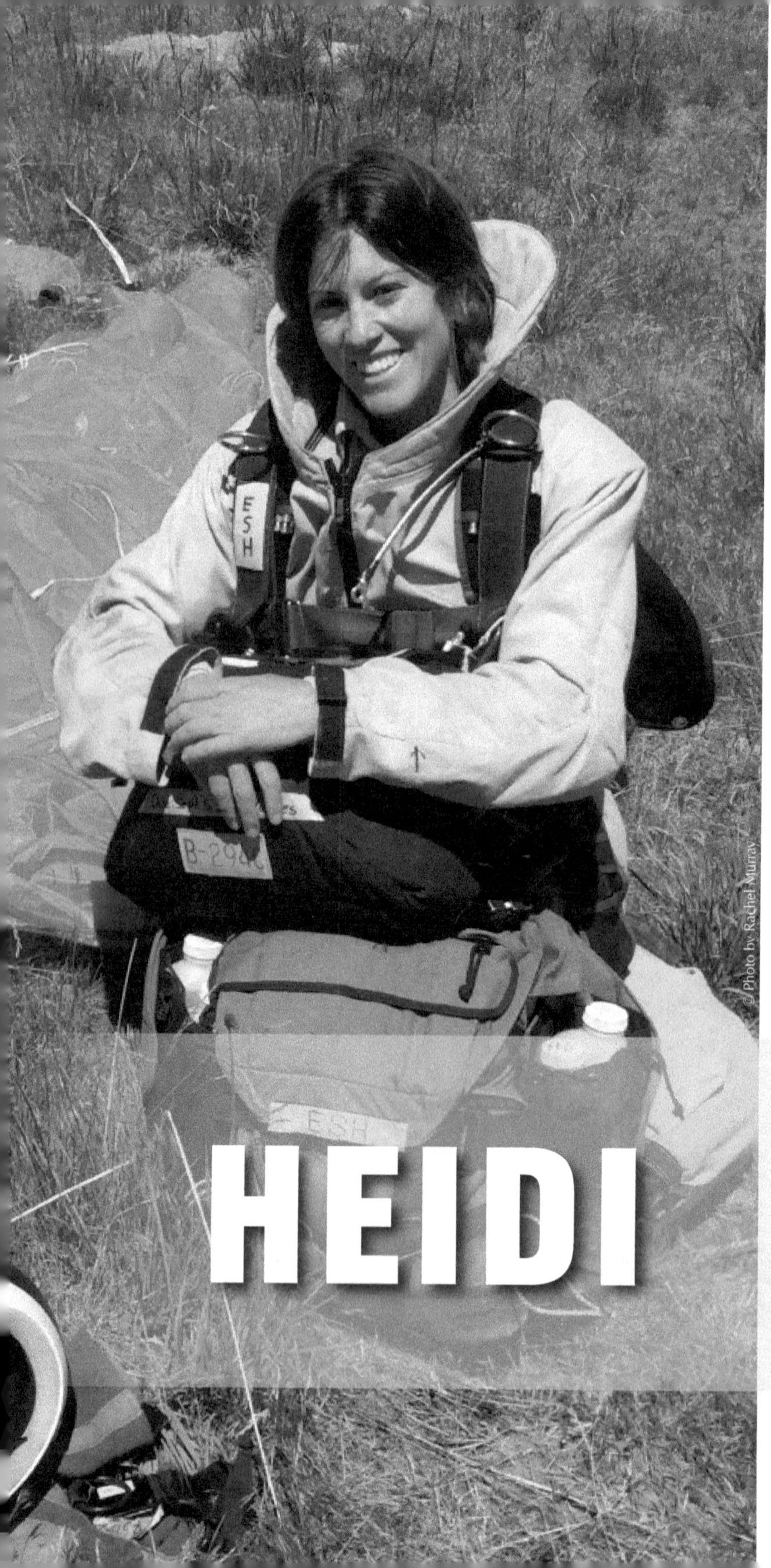

© Photo by Rachel Murray

HEIDI IS QUIET. People often ask me what she's like. A bulldog. She has a bite. She is relentless. Like others in the world of firefighting, she has grit—the kind you aren't born with. She had to earn it. In a realm dominated by males, this physically small and quiet female stands out. And boy, does she stand out!

Recently I checked on Heidi, and she texted me back referring to herself as a "muscly hamster," complete with a gif of a cute little rodent snatching a tiny barbell. It made me laugh—the silly image of Heidi as a hamster. She has a sense of humor that sneaks up on you. She is one of the physically smallest females that I have coached, but don't let that distract from who she really is and what she has accomplished. She was the first female smokejumper candidate that I had the pleasure of preparing for smokejumper rookie training, which is one of the most competitive and physically rigorous training processes out there. Imagine Navy Seals, but instead of BUDS candidates carrying boats and logs, smokejumper rookies are tested and trained in the mountains at elevation with running, rucking, and hard PT (physical training), followed by a crash course in parachuting protocols.

Before I tell the full story of Heidi, I must begin... at my beginning. I was born in Chicago, moved to Sedona, Arizona, when I was nine where I grew up through high school, and ended up moving further west for college to play football and run track at the University of Redlands in Southern California. After three years of football, four years of track and field, and two individual national championship wins (decathlon, 2007, and long jump, 2008), I graduated with a bachelors in studio art (ceramics and sculpture), and a master's degree in higher education (which allowed me to continue training for track and field while I was in grad school). After college, I wanted to continue training for the Olympic Trials, so I packed up and drove from Redlands to Champaign-Urbana, a small town in the middle of the Central Illinois cornfields. That's where I began my coaching career. I started as an unpaid volunteer assistant track and field coach at the University of Illinois in Champaign-Urbana. I loved living there—by day, aspiring Olympian decathlete; by afternoon, track coach; and at night, to make ends meet, a server dressed in all black at a small Italian restaurant in downtown Champaign called Manzella's Italian Patio. Ironically, the place did not have a patio. I met some good friends there, and we had a great time in the Champaign area. If you have never worked in the service industry, let me tell you a secret: they like to party. Even though I was training diligently during the week, on the weekends, it was too enticing to pass up a party with the Manzella's gang. After closing the restaurant, we often hit downtown or campus town HARD, bitching about the evening's toughest customers, and the server who received the lowest tip from a table that evening had to take a shot of Malört. Ahh, to be young again.

It was at Illinois that I first fell in love with coaching female athletes. Don't get me wrong. In the past 14 years, I have had rewarding experiences and coaching success with male teams and athletes, both at Illinois and afterwards. But for me, there is something uniquely rewarding about helping a woman train to conquer colossal goals. The stakes seem higher, the physicality more challenging, and the success at the end, sweeter. It feels like I'm a distant supporting actor in the heroic battle story of David and Goliath, except David's name was Heidi, and then Sierra, and then Cam. From my experience, females often don't bring as much ego into the coach-athlete relationship, and yet they remain fiercely competitive. Women also seem to place more trust in me than my male athletes. That could just be my perception. However, when time is of the essence, there is no room for battling egos. Especially in cases like Heidi's, where we had less than six months to prepare her for competing with males in the physical prime of their lives to become smokejumpers.

I was extremely fortunate to begin my coaching career at what felt like the apex of the collegiate coaching world, Division I, in the Big Ten Conference. As an Illini volunteer assistant coach (and eventually a modestly paid assistant coach), I had the honor and pleasure to learn from two world-class coaches. The lessons gleaned from Tonja Buford-Bailey and Mike Erb in the Armory (Illinois' massive indoor track and training facility), at the outdoor track, and trekking for hours across the country in buses, vans, and planes laid the foundation of my coaching and professional life and continue to guide me to this day. Without them, the events that led to the writing of this book would not have happened.

Tonja Buford-Bailey was the most decorated female track and field sprinter and hurdler to ever run at Illinois. She accumulated more Big Ten Conference championship event wins than anyone in the school's history (25 individual Big Ten titles—that means she won 25 individual events at the Big Ten indoor and outdoor championships during her 4 years as a collegiate athlete). Eventually she competed in three Olympics, winning a bronze medal in the 400 hurdles at the 1996 Olympic Games in Atlanta, Georgia, and breaking the 400m hurdles world record (losing that same race by a single hundredth of a second), but she never received the recognition that she deserved. Turns out that people don't remember the second-place finisher even if they broke the world record. Tonja now coaches an all-black female track and field super-team in Austin, Texas, a team chock full of champions on the world stage. This group might have more track and field national and international medals than any other team on the planet. I could write an entire chapter on Tonja, and a better writer could fill a book.

I shadowed under Tonja for three seasons at Illinois. She taught me how to keep athletes humble. If an athlete's ego began to run wild, she would text the athlete to come to her office, sit them down, and straighten them out, not letting them budge an inch. If two athletes had interpersonal issues, Tonja would call both athletes into her office, and they'd hash it out until a solution was reached. Sometimes she let me sit in on these meetings. I had never in my life seen someone take care of drama so efficiently and effectively. She was also an incredibly intuitive coach. Sure, she had season plans and a general sense of which direction she was going to take her athletes and at what pace, but if she felt something needed changing during a training block, training week, individual training session, or even a single drill within a training session, Tonja would make changes on the fly, and they always seemed dead-on. Her intuition led the female Illini track and field team to a Big Ten Championship win in 2013.

On that coaching staff at Illinois, Mike Erb was also my college track coach. That was my "in" to train and coach at Illinois after college. Mike was still a young coach when I worked under him, and nowadays, he cringes at some of the training methods that he relied upon to prepare me and other jumpers, throwers, and multi-event athletes early on in his career, but I still absorbed the majority of my coaching knowledge through interacting with Mike, reading books he recommended, and going with him to coaching seminars and conferences. Mike taught me how to plan with technical specificity. At the beginning of each season, we would sit down in front of a large white board, and together we sketched out the season. His method was to start at the end, at the culmination event, and work backwards logically and tediously. I used this method with Heidi. Through working alongside Mike (and from running as an athlete under his coaching), I also learned how to get into an athlete's head.

I distinctly remember competing at decathlons with Mike coaching me. He only let me know what I needed to be successful. He knew that I was a data freak, and my mind would run wild if I had a look at the points or knew how the decathlon scoring system worked, so he never taught me. This allowed him to use other "carrots" to motivate me during each of the ten events within each decathlon. He knew that I was competitive, so he would pick different athletes for me to contest with during specific events. He might say, "You need to beat that guy in the high jump. That'll put you right where you need to be," or "look at him, he's weaker than you. You will eat him alive in the 400m. Don't let him think for even a second that he can hang."

Sometimes I entered large competitions with a meek attitude, and these ego-boosting comments and athlete-targets helped me focus. He also helped me downregulate. At a moment's notice, if he sensed that I was too amped up, he would inject calmness to help bring me back down to earth. "Go hide out somewhere and focus on your chi gong or something," he would advise knowing that I threw the discus better when I was calm.

From Mike, I learned to read athletes, first with watching how he coached me, and then I began to watch closely how he worked with others who had different personality types. Eventually, at Illinois, he let me work solely with a few challenging athletes at big competitions to let me learn on the fly. Perhaps the most important thing he taught me was how to leverage mental training strategies like imagery and breathwork to improve the quality of my mindset. I think these strategies helped Heidi the most.

In 2011, after my final season coaching at Illinois, I had limited coaching job offers from some mid-major division I universities in small Midwest towns. The jobs paid little, and I don't think that Jessica, my girlfriend at the time, would have followed me to one of those towns. In fact, when I asked her how she felt about me moving away to coach at one of those universities, she replied, "If you do that, you're stupid." She always had a way with words. I still don't know if she meant I would be stupid for moving to those small towns, or for moving away from her.

I knew I was falling in love with Jessica about six months before. We had met up for a long, fast run through the forest together. She was the first girl who could keep up with me, physically and metaphorically. During the run, I probably said something odd, and she asked me if I was a serial killer, and I said yes, that I had dug a hole for her and it was up ahead. Jess and I have been together for 12 years now, 5 of them as husband and wife. We still joke about killing each other. The hole is still just around the corner.

Jessica and I met at the grand re-opening of a bar called The White Horse, which everyone in town called "white ho," which has been previously shut down for "renovations" (ahem ... underage drinking). We were each there with different groups of friends, and at the end of the night, as I scanned the place for my friends, I locked eyes with a beautiful, tall, strong, and kind-looking redhead smiling at me from the other side of the bar. I had, as most young males do, an irrational fear of red-headed women, for they are rare. So, naturally, I was terrified of her. Who knew what existed beyond that innocent smile and those tight jeans? I thought it would be interesting to find out, so I mustered up some courage and walked over to her. "Are you smiling at me?" I asked. She laughed, pulled her hair to the other side of her neck, and said, "I like tall guys, and you look nice. Also, I'm here with a guy friend who is hammered and getting creepy." I was sober because it was Thursday, and I had heavy training the next day, so I offered to drive her home. She didn't live far. When we arrived at her apartment, she invited me in, and we sat on the couch and talked about life for a long time. It got late, so I told her I had to train early in the morning. She walked me to the door, we said goodbye, and as the door closed, I said goodbye and she said, "See you never..."

Instead of pursuing one of those mid-major track coaching positions and moving away from Jessica, I took a one-year hiatus from coaching and accepted a corporate job at a start-up company selling spinal medical devices in the Chicago area. I moved back in with my parents and saved up money for one year. Jessica graduated from Illinois with a degree in Integrative Biology and moved back home to live with her folks. We did the distance thing for that entire year. Near the end of that year in the spine industry, I disliked what was happening to my body and mind. I had become quick to anger and was gaining some fluff around my mid-section. I also took a look around at the older men within my profession and decided that I needed a change. They were ruthlessly competitive, which I liked, but they also seemed unhappy, unhealthy, and stressed. I didn't want to end up like them.

When I got a call to move across the country for a coaching position at a CrossFit gym in my college town, I jumped at the opportunity. I gave my two weeks' notice and drove to California the following week. Convincing Jessica to move with me was tough. At the last minute, she decided to join me after talking with her best friend and realizing that she had nothing to gain if she stayed in Illinois, and she'd lose me if she didn't come with me.

We arrived by car in the summer of 2012. We drove separately, her in a little forest green 2000 Chevy Cavalier, and me in a 2002 white Chevy Malibu. To help pass the time, we each brought a riding buddy. I rode with Mike, and Jess rode with a friend from college. During the last hour of our drive through the city of Indio to our destination town of Redlands, as the August sun beat down on the road and the temperature soared above 110, Jess stopped sweating. She didn't know this was a bad thing at the time. Her poor little car didn't have A/C (for the record, my A/C didn't work so well, either). When we arrived at our destination of Redlands, California, I directed our caravan to Heska's, my favorite sandwich shop from college. That day, the heat wave which baked our cars had also knocked the power out all over Southern California. All we wanted was a cold drink, and we couldn't even get that. And then Jess fainted.

We almost called the ambulance, but Jess's friend was a travel nurse and helped orchestrate hydration and cooling for the next hour or so until Jess was lucid enough to leave. What an entrance into town. I don't think that Jessica ever forgave Redlands for that rough encounter. First impressions are lasting, as they say.

We had moved into an area of California that people call the I.E., short for the Inland Empire, which sits about an hour east of L.A. and an hour west of Palm Springs. The I.E. is an area brimming with non-functional lifted trucks and low profile Honda Civics with the catalytic converters either stolen or removed on purpose to make them louder, a plethora of tramp stamps, tribal tattoos, fake breasts, oversized sunglasses, Dickies, wallet chains, and palm trees (which aren't even native to the area) with dead leaves on them. All of this sits atop an arid desert that smells like dead fish for a month out of the year when the wind blows from the Salton Sea and bakes under the desert sun in our smog-filled valley. Some days, you can't even see the massive San Bernardino mountains through the haze. I loved it.

And right in the middle of this desolate expanse rests my college town. Ahh, good old Redlands. This small, upscale city defiantly sits juxtaposed to the surrounding I.E. I loved driving through the green rolling hills filled with historic Craftsman homes and hidden hillside mansions. It felt like I was living in a Bruce Springsteen song. The sunsets can also be quite lovely through the haze. I still miss this little town. I made friendships here that may never be surpassed in the rest of my life.

After taking the weekend to unpack, I immediately began working at the CrossFit gym. It was at this gym where Heidi and I first met. We had both attended the University of Redlands and even graduated in the same year, but our paths rarely crossed. At the CrossFit gym, we interacted through group classes, which means our time working together was limited at best. I do remember that she had quite an engine, and her calisthenic endurance was impressive. Little did I know that our interactions here would lead to a relationship that would change my life forever.

Work at the gym was tough. The days were long, split shifts starting at 4:30 a.m. and ending at 8 p.m. each weekday with a midday break lasting a couple of hours. I spent my breaks with Jessica—training, eating, and sometimes napping. Weekend classes put me in the gym from 5:30 a.m. to noon on Saturdays, and a Sunday class at 10:00 a.m. Since I was the new guy, I frequently worked 7 days a week.

On top of the difficulties from my intense coaching schedule, Jessica was completely new to California. She didn't know anyone. She didn't know her way around. No job. She had never lived outside of Illinois. She grew up in a small farm town west of Chicago with a population of two thousand people—complete with two bars, a Subway sandwich shop, and miles of cornfields. To say our first few months living in Redlands were rough on the relationship is an understatement. We barely made it through. I don't know what I would have done without Jessica there, though. She didn't like my gym and signed up for a different gym across town. When my boss found out, he threatened to fire me if I didn't get Jess back at our gym. He even offered to comp her membership and those of her new friends at the other gym. I told him to fire me then, and he did.

A few weeks passed, and the whole time I wondered what I was going to do. I called Mike and Tonja, and each of them got their feelers out for track coaching positions around the country. When I told Jess we might have to move to Texas for a track coaching job, she said she wasn't going to move again and was going to move back home. I consoled her and said we'd stay in Redlands. That's when Jess said she'd introduce me to Chad, the owner of her new gym. I met him and we got along well. That weekend, he invited us to join in a little get-together at his house on a Sunday morning after some 5k that his gym members were participating in. A gathering on a Sunday morning sounded innocent enough.

Apparently, people at this gym liked to party. By noon, we were all stinking, stammering, stumbling drunk. Everyone. It was unreal. I distinctly remember standing in the back yard in just my underwear, overhead squatting a 200-pound brick of a kid named Sutton. Halfway out of the bottom of the squat, I lost my balance and dropped him on top of me, landing in a pile with hysterical laughter from us and the dozen spectators.

After that day, Chad offered me a job. I gladly accepted and remained there coaching and learning from him and our staff during the next five years. We never had a party like that again. Eventually, Chad entrusted me to run much of the training and coaching, so I had more freedom to coach the members how I wanted. I modeled my coaching style after Mike and Tonja, where I learned the theoretical and interpersonal aspects of coaching. It was at CrossFit South Redlands where I grew my base of experience, coaching over thirty-five classes a week. It became my "testing lab." In the early days, everything was experimental. Nowadays, training *still* feels somewhat experimental because I'm always searching for a better way. However, after a few successes, I started to believe in myself and began to move past the youthful, idealistic belief that I knew everything.

Within a couple of years of coaching at the new spot, I began to think about the future. How would I progress my career? Open my own gym? Who would go to it? I had some coaching experience, but that didn't seem like enough to set myself apart. I decided that I needed more school! I already had one master's degree (that I didn't yet use professionally). Why not get another one, but this time make it more applicable to coaching!

I looked up master's programs and found a hybrid program that was part online and part in-person. The school was Southern Utah University in Cedar City, Utah. That was only about 6 hours from Redlands. I checked the program reviews and was impressed by the student outcomes. I also talked to a program graduate, and he was reassuring about the program's quality. He said the education he received at SUU was excellent, highlighted the small cohort size, and painted the program as an opportunity to get to know the instructors well. I signed up, excited for who I would become over the next few years of school.

Even though I worked under great coaches in the track and field realm, up until this point, I had little experience creating my own training programs. At Illinois, Tonja and Mike had created the track and field technical training, and the athletes usually did well. All I had to do was show up and coach their technique, following the training that was written for the day. Mike and I wrote the strength training for our field and multi-event athletes. The most hands-on programming experience was given to me by Tonja. She allowed me to write much of the strength training for her sprinters and hurdlers. I also taught the women how to perform the Olympic lifts.

Over the three seasons that I worked under Tonja and Mike, the University of Illinois Track and Field program created multiple Big Ten Conference champions, broke some school and conference records, performed well at the regional championships, and even produced some nationally competitive athletes and relay teams, and a national champion hurdler. A handful of these athletes went on to compete professionally.

In the years after coaching these athletes, under Tonja's guidance, some went on to the Olympic Trials, World Championships, and the Olympics. One of our Illini female sprinters who also threw shot put (an insanely rare combination at the division I level, especially considering she was a Big Ten finalist in both) earned a medal at the Olympics in Bobsled! While these athletes were in college training with me, I felt like I helped with those wins, but it never felt like my work. I was always a support coach, an assistant to the decision makers. Heidi was my first opportunity to test my ability without anyone else's influence, guided by the coaching lessons gleaned from Tonja and Mike.

It had been a few years since I last saw or heard from Heidi. One day, she texted me out of the blue and asked to speak with me. She mentioned that she ran into Emily Elliott, an athlete of mine who I was training for the California's Strongest Female, a strongman competition which took place each year near Huntington Beach. Emily and Heidi knew each other from that first CrossFit gym, and Heidi stated that she was looking for someone to train her for something big. I had helped prepare Emily to win California's Strongest lightweight female the year before, and she had good things to say about my coaching and programming and had passed my number to Heidi. The connection was made. It was time to chat.

WEDNESDAY OCTOBER 12, 2016 (INITIAL PHONE CALL)

Before we began working together, I knew that Heidi was some type of firefighter; I just didn't know *what kind*. Hell, I didn't even know that there *were* different kinds. I thought if a building catches fire, the fire department shows up, rescues babies and dogs, sprays it down with hoses, and the heroes get pictured in the paper. I guess that's kind of true, but firefighting is also so much more—specifically, wildland firefighting.

Heidi and I planned a time to talk, and I offered to call her. She waved me off and said she'd call me. It felt like she wanted to remain in control. I had time midday between my split shift at the second CrossFit gym, and that's when we planned to talk. She called and we spoke. Heidi has a soft and high-pitched voice. Her manner of speaking is straightforward and stoic. Militaristic. I have come to learn that Heidi goes out and gets what she wants. She calls the shots. She is sweet and sincere about it, too. Along with the soft impression that I initially experienced from her, there is a directness and stubbornness that has allowed her to accomplish many great things.

Since we didn't really know each other too well, and it had been years since we last saw each other, we small talked for an instant, followed by silence, and then she asked me to train her for smokejumping. I had not heard of this profession before.

Before I could ask questions, as many in the military or wildland fire will do, Heidi went off on a tangent that was clear to her and murky at best to me, the story filled with wildland firefighting industry jargon and bases and excitement and adventure. I hung on as best I could until she finished. Essentially, Heidi wanted to go jump out of an airplane to fight forest fires. This is called smokejumping. Apparently, it is a thing people do. Also apparently, it's very difficult to make it through rookie training, the prerequisite physical training to prepare smokejumpers for the demands of the job.

> In the years since this encounter, after working with a dozen wildland firefighters, I realize the tone in elite fire is similar to military special ops. They seem to exist on another plane of life where only the most dangerous experiences rev them up, and through everything else, they remain cool as a James Dean cucumber. Consider this later in the book when I discuss Performance Arousal Theory.

At the time, I had no idea about how someone would become a smokejumper. With my full-time job coaching and growing part-time gig programming for athletes, I didn't have time to look up the nuances. I barely knew what questions to ask Heidi to best prepare her.

Years later, I finally learned about the application process to become a smokejumper. The process is stringent and takes anywhere from 3-6 months, sometimes years for applicants to earn a candidate offer. Bases desire experienced wildland firefighters with leadership experience. To be competitive, attractive applicants have 4+ years of wildland fire experience. Leadership can be demonstrated by being a squad boss on a hotshot crew or a task leader on a fire. Bases also consider other leadership experiences outside of fire, but wildland fire experience is weighted more heavily in the selection process. The application process varies by base. Generally, the paperwork portion of the application process takes 3-6 weeks. Applicants fill out a government job application (BLM and USFS are government positions), submit a 3-part resume, and wait for interview calls. For strong candidates, supervisory reference checks are conducted. Usually, younger firefighters work with veterans who help them through the long and confusing governmental application process. If you screw up the application, you are not considered.

To learn about this process, I spoke to Matt Bowers, a retired 27-year smokejumper veteran who completed his tenure as Crew Supervisor (2nd in command behind the Base Supervisor) at the Boise Smokejumper Base. He oversaw hiring, rookie training, conduct, and jumper performance. He even held the position of rookie trainer in the early 2000s for two years.

Rookie trainers are complete badasses. Heidi said that her rookie trainers at Boise "looked like Spartans," and a few of them had scored a perfect 400 points on the PT test, meaning they could perform 25+ strict pull-ups, 120+ push-ups, 150+ sit-ups in 3 minutes, and run a sub-8:00 mile and a half (5:20

mile pace). Consider that rookie trainers must accompany the rookies everywhere they go for 40–50 hours a week for 5–6 weeks in a row. If the rookies run a half marathon on a cold and rainy Tuesday morning in April, the rookie trainers are running alongside them. Matt Bowers must have been a machine in 2003.

Matt said they'd interview 1/3 of the qualified applicants out of the 100 or so that applied each year. Next, the base hires 6–12 rookies. Once the candidate offer is accepted by the rookie, their contract with the base hinges on their passing rookie training. I smiled when I learned that rookie training is not a selection process. For all these years, after coaching many wildland fire athletes, I had thought rookie training was designed to separate the wheat from the chaff, revealing physically talented and team-oriented smokejumpers. I was incorrect.

Bases spend a ton of time, money, and resources finding and hiring rookies that they hope are a good fit. Matt actually said he'd love it if everyone made it through. But that's not reality. Out of the average 8 rookies that undergo rookie training, 4–6 of them graduate.

In 2022, there were about 400 smokejumpers across nine total bases in the Pacific Northwestern United States. There are two BLM bases (Fairbanks, Alaska; Boise, Idaho), and seven USFS Bases (Grangeville, Idaho; Missoula, Montana; Redding, California; Redmond, Oregon; Northern California Smokejumpers; West Yellowstone, Montana; and McCall, Idaho). Out of those 9 bases, there are about 12 female smokejumpers.

Smokejumping began more than 80 years ago in the 1940s to combat wildfires in a novel and innovative way. It took 40 years for the first female to earn a smokejumper position. In 1979, the first female smokejumper, Deanne Schulman, passed the physical standards of rookie training but was washed due to being a few pounds under the required weight. At the time, it was known there were men at other smokejumper bases who were also underweight, so Deanne filed an Equal Employment Opportunity Commission complaint, which was supported by one of those underweight men, and Deanne was cleared to attempt rookie training again the next year if she weighed at least 130 pounds on the first day of rookie training. The following year, she made weight and subsequently passed rookie training.

Since then, the required bodyweight has been lowered to 120 pounds, but the physical standards for the run, pull-ups, push-ups, sit-ups, and the 110-pound pack test remain the same, albeit faster. Shulman completed the pack test in over three hours. Heidi would have to perform this challenge significantly faster.

To become part of this special breed of firefighters, Heidi needed to pass rookie training. She informed me that she had failed twice during the previous two seasons, and this year, she was pursuing one final attempt in the upcoming spring season. It was currently October, and rookie training would begin in mid-April. She chose me to help her prepare.

I remember being nervous on the phone. Jess and I only ran the A/C when it was really hot, so this morning it was off, and today was looking to be over 80; it was only 10:30 am, but I was already sweating as I sat at my large kitchen table which was way too big for my tiny ground floor apartment.

Heidi talked about standards: mindset, strengths, and weaknesses. She spoke of the different smokejumping bases across the country. She chose to attempt rookie training at Boise because it was a difficult base to rookie out of. Rookie training at Bureau of Land Management bases tend to have a lower passing rate than the US Forest Service bases. I asked Matt Bowers if BLM bases are more challenging to rookie at, and he laughed, "All the bases are tough."

In the 1990's, the entire smokejumper employment roster at the Boise Smokejumper Base was comprised of 80% transfers. Yep, 8 out of every 10 employees had rookied elsewhere and transferred in. This was initially driven by three factors. One, in the 1990s, BLM bases offered more enticing benefits than US Forest Service bases. Second, some employees at BLM bases were offered year-round employment, which was extremely attractive compared to USFS jumpers who worked almost exclusively as seasonal employees. And third, rookies washed out of Boise in droves. Nowadays, the USFS also offers comparable benefits and some year-round positions, but the legacy about the difficulty of rookie training at Boise and Fairbanks has survived.

As Heidi flowed on with her fire-jargon-fueled, stream-of-consciousness information dump, I took notes in a spiral notebook as fast as I could while trying to keep up as she mainlined her laundry list of physical, mental, and emotional needs for rookie training into my brain. Once she finished, she asked, "What do you think?" Overwhelmed with questions and the sheer mag-nitude of her quest, the perspiration I was already experiencing increased. I thought that she was crazy. I left my first thought in my head and my ques-tions for our next conversation.

"Sounds exciting! I'd love to work with you," I chimed, feeling the tug of adventure at this opportunity to help her accomplish something challeng-ing and awesome. I also want to prove to myself that I could take an athlete and mold them into what they wanted to be, from start to finish. No outside influences. No overseers. My first solo athlete! To end our first wild ride of a conversation, in a sweet and genuine voice brimming with hope, Heidi asked, "Do you think it's possible?" And with the unearned confidence supported by inexperience and a touch of naivety, I replied, "Yeah! Let's find out."

PLANNING FOR HEIDI

Heidi already had a few years of wildland fire experience. She had worked on many different wildland crews: engine, rappelling, helitack, and hotshot. For most wildland fire employees, the occupation is seasonal, spanning April or

May through September or October. After the season, they take the late fall and winter seasons off and return in the spring. Over the years, Heidi had climbed the ranks and was a senior firefighter. She worked year-round.

She would prepare each off-season for the busy wildfire season ahead by training towards top physical shape. Wildland firefighters take the physicality and mortal dangers of their careers very seriously, and they train hard to prepare for the dangers ahead. After washing out of smokejumper rookie training the previous two seasons, Heidi worked on Boise's helitack crew.

Wildland firefighting consists of several different groups including hand crews, engine crews, fuel crews, hotshots, helitack, wildland fire modules, rappelers, and smokejumpers (that list is in order of experience and difficulty). Smokejumpers parachute out of planes to prevent forest fires from spreading. They are an elite branch of wildland firefighters who are called in, often first (along with helitack crews), and often for small forest fires that start from lightning strikes and other natural and sometimes unnatural means. They work in crews and jump out of nine different bases scattered around the West Coast and the Pacific Northwest: California, Idaho, Montana, Oregon, Washington, and Alaska.

Wildland firefighters are a different breed. In the off-season when they take time off from fighting forest fires all over the western US, many seem to travel the world chasing adventure. Extreme in their careers, they also seem to push the limits in their personal lives outside of work. They might backcountry skin up a remote snow-covered mountain for hours just to ski down a few times. They sportfish and spearfish and free dive. They run marathons and ultramarathons. They might pace-set for their older brother on 64 miles of a 100-mile ultramarathon, at elevation through rough terrain. They seek adrenaline as much in the off-season as they do during the fire season—where they might hike towards a massive forest fire carrying 80–120 pounds of gear and supplies on their back, wielding chain saws and other fire suppressant equipment, cut line for hours into the night, and then high tail it back out again before sunrise when the wind shift brings the blaze right to their flank.

> Backcountry skinning is attaching synthetic "skins" onto the bottom of cross-country skis to increase grip while hiking up a mountain to ski down the ungroomed and potentially treacherous backcountry terrain.

My first week working directly with Heidi was underway. We had planned to work almost completely remotely. I spoke to her on Wednesday, and then spent the rest of the week brainstorming and drafting her program. Heidi was a bit busted up from the previous fire season. The fire seasons always wipe firefighters out physically, and they often take a month or two off from physical training to allow their bodies and minds to recover before they begin physical preparation for the next season.

Heidi didn't have that luxury. We only had six months to train, and she needed every week of that time to prepare. To get her moving initially, I wrote her a very easy first week of training to feel out the waters. I had only coached her in a group format before, and many years ago, so this initial period was important for me to learn what Heidi could handle, and at what rate of increase I could push her with minimal risk.

Heidi's main limitation after her most recent fire season was plantar fasciitis. Plantar Fasciitis is often experienced as heel pain or pain along the arch of the foot. This condition is caused by inflammation of the plantar fascia, the thick band of connective tissue that links the ball of foot with the heal along the sole of the foot.

Years earlier, I had experienced this persistent and nagging foot pain when competing as a track athlete in college. It lasted for years and finally dissipated after I began training without shoes. For Heidi, we began adding in barefoot training slowly and followed up each session with a "foot care" regimen during which Heidi would first roll the arches of her feet out with a PVC pipe or lacrosse ball, and then would stretch her calves and foam roll her shins. This was her primary method of lower leg mobility and tissue work, and after this, she would work further up her legs on her hamstrings, quadriceps, glutes, and hip flexors. Along with foot and ankle strengthening, I strongly felt this approach would help her heal, so I wrote it into her training from the beginning and taught her how to care for her feet and lower legs.

My master's program was almost complete! I was taking my final class, a thesis support course, taught by Dr. Camille Thomas. I chose her to chair my thesis because she had critiqued my work mercilessly in previous courses. The week after starting up with Heidi, I had a conversation with Dr. Thomas. There were some data transfer issues with some of my tables in my thesis, and she was helping me troubleshoot. I was glad to have her in my corner, but she was tough on me. From grammar to content to formatting my tables, she wouldn't let me slide an inch. She was a perfect match for me. For the previous two years, I had been working through Southern Utah University's Master of Science program in Sport Conditioning and Performance. The classes were often in alignment with my professional work, which I found inspiring. It was refreshing to apply concepts learned in class directly to athletes at the gym that same day, and now I could apply my lessons to developing Heidi.

The combination of working hard on my thesis, and at the same time crafting Heidi's programming was a perfect storm of knowledge and inspiration. I began to subconsciously look for solutions to some of Heidi's training concerns in my master's thesis research. Taking Heidi's case was beginning to light a fire under my ass after many months of dragging slowly through the painstakingly tedious thesis editing process.

After spending time each day working on my thesis, when it was time, to shift gears to programming, I had to put the thesis to rest before clearing mental space for Heidi. She was a new type of athlete that I had not coached before, so it took me a lot of time to research and prepare for creating her program. I started with her previous experience at the two rookie trainings and then began to weave in my own training knowledge.

Heidi said that smokejumper rookie training was the most difficult thing she had ever attempted. She had gone through some rough physical training experiences while on hotshot crews, but nothing else had compared. The physical, mental, and psychological challenges were insane. Before she could even apply to become a smokejumper, she had to show that she was made of the "right stuff" by working in wildland fire for years. The bases that had hired her thought she was worth a shot, but she had not yet proven physically ready for the job demands.

While working with Heidi, the smokejumper application and hiring process were not yet known to me, so we stuck to focusing strictly on the physical demands. That is where my expertise resides. She listed a few dozen things that she would need to accomplish and a handful of mental considerations that would be useful as well. The basic requirements are passing the smokejumper PT Test (short for Physical Training Test) that hold minimum acceptable performance standards of pull-ups, push-ups, sit-ups, 1.5-mile run, and a pack test. Failure to meet the minimum standards at any point during rookie training prompts immediate dismissal. The slang for this is washing out. BLM

Rookie Training PT* Test Requirements (*PT stands for Physical Training)

Heidi chose the Boise Smokejumper Base to undergo rookie training. The Boise Base falls under the Bureau of Land Management (BLM), and the ***minimum*** physical standards they test on the first day of rookie training are:

- Run 1.5 miles in 10:47
- 6 pull-ups
- 30 push-ups
- Pack test - carry a 110-pound pack for 3 miles in under 65 minutes

The BLM Smokejumpers also have established minimum "High Standards," suggesting that these marks are a good indication of an individual's potential for successful completion of rookie training:

- Run 1.5 miles in 9:30 or run 3 miles in 22:30
- 10 pull-ups
- 35 push-ups
- 60 sit-ups
- Pack test - carry a 110-pound pack for 3 miles in under 65 minutes

Heidi's initial goals were more aggressive in everything but the pack test:

- Run 1.5 miles in 9:00
- 20 pull-ups
- 85 push-ups
- 130 sit-ups
- Pack test - carry a 110-pound pack for 3 miles in under 65 minutes

smokejumper bases have "High Standards," which are even higher performance metrics than the USFS. Failure to meet the minimum high standards is grounds for immediate washing at BLM bases.

Heidi had six months to train. In my mind, she was a professional athlete, and I treated her like one. She had no job to bog her down and no boyfriend to distract her. She was ready for full training mode. I could write her 8 hours of training each day, and she would have the time to complete it. This was so freeing for me! It seemed like the only restrictions were her own physical limits, which I intended to explore. And from what I knew of her character, if I wrote her 8 hours of training, she'd get it done, no questions asked. No complaining. Even to her detriment. This was a blessing and a curse.

To be successful, we both knew that we had to push her beyond where she had gone physically and mentally before. To attain her goals this time around, she would have to show up to rookie training a different athlete entirely. A different person. Her best marks were already impressive, but Heidi wanted to arrive light-years beyond her physical self from last year to show the rookie trainers that she was more ready than ever. The higher her initial performances in rookie training, the better, so long as that didn't sacrifice performance later during the following weeks.

In 2015, Heidi was hired as a smokejumper for McCall. During this first attempt at smokejumper rookie training, she washed out in week four due to "unsatisfactory Exits and PLFs" (PLFs are Parachute Landing Falls, a crucial element to safe parachute landings while smokejumping). Rookie trainers must prepare rookies for the job, and when they spot dangerous patterns or physical weakness, they wash the rookie for their own safety and the safety of the entire crew. Sending an unfit smokejumper into a forest fire could prove severe or deadly for everyone involved.

Even though washing Heidi was the right thing for the rookie trainers to do that year, it was disheartening because she had passed the physical requirements and made it through the first three hellacious weeks. However, her physical strength and endurance were not high enough to allow optimal physical and cognitive functioning in those later weeks of training. This led to her mind faltering, and she made mistakes on the jump tower.

In 2016, during her second attempt, this time at Boise, she washed out on day one. Last year at McCall, she passed the 110-pound pack test, coming in just under the 90-minute time cap. This time around, at Boise, she failed the same test because on BLM bases, the time cap is 65 minutes. Damn those High Standards! It was simply too heavy for her to carry at that pace. This year, her plan was to arrive at rookie training with all her weaknesses shored up, especially the heavy pack.

Heidi was 34 at the time, which one might think is too old for smokejumping considering the physical demands of rookie training and the job itself. Add in that she is five-foot-two, one hundred and fifteen pounds. Many of the rookies who would be competing against her are twenty- to thirty-year-old males brimming with peak hormones. However, Heidi was driven, committed, and relentless in pursuit of her goal. Two failures over the previous two jump seasons did not deter her from a third attempt (because she's crazy—her words).

From her past two failed rookie trainings, Heidi had some knowledge of what to expect, and we relied on this to plan our attack. However, the element of the unknown is always a strong factor in any rookie training, including smokejumping.

During the planning phase, Heidi provided me with what tasks and standards she thought she would need to perform and strategically layered together training to address all the demands. Over the coming months, my plan was to build volume with each of the specific tasks that Heidi deemed worthy of her training time.

Years ago, before working with Heidi and other female athletes like her, I, as most others, held limited beliefs and had no idea that females COULD do something like this. Of course, they can. It's very simple. They would have to hack it, both physically and mentally, just as well as the men and other female rookies in their class.

Because of my personality and youth, babying my athletes was one of my biggest limitations as a coach—letting someone take an easier route than they should for fear of breaking them (or losing them as a client or friend). Perhaps this comes from my own athletic experience. I know what it feels like to train at a high level and to break. I have physically broken a few times. And I know what fifteen-plus weekly hours of intense training, six days a week for many months on end does to the body and to the mind.

In college, I had a couple of serious girlfriends, and when I neared the peak of my training each season, I was not emotionally available for them because I was barely holding on psychologically myself. This caused relationship problems ending in heartbreak, which put that much more pressure on me during big competitions. Heavy training takes a significant toll. It exacerbates and magnifies everything in your life. Perhaps I allowed this to make me too empathetic.

To snap me out of it, Heidi highlighted the repercussions for under-preparation in her notes on how to prepare her. She experienced physical under-preparation, which caused the memorization of complex and specific jump protocols to become increasingly challenging for her, and she washed out of rookie training. If you don't get rolled for physically not being able to hack it, they can roll you for mentally not being able to hack it as well. Take a closer look at that sequence. The mental breakdown is initiated by physical fatigue. Showing up physically prepared with a high tolerance for the unknowns that she'd undergo would allow for optimal mental performance when required to learn and execute new tasks with proficiency through heavy fatigue. Heidi was determined to do everything she could this time around to be successful—or die trying.

SUNDAY OCTOBER 23, 2016
(INITIAL PLANNING, 27 WEEKS OUT, JUST OVER SIX MONTHS)

Since first speaking with Heidi, I had been turning over programming structure and planning ideas in my head. It was becoming difficult to concentrate on my master's thesis. I sat at my big kitchen table with an 18 x 24-inch sketch pad left over from my days in college as an art student, and I drafted out a half week of initial training for Heidi, just to get her moving. I planned to write her a full week of training during the coming weekend when I had more time.

I considered that she was fresh out of her most recent fire season when she had been working on the helitack crew, so she was physically fatigued and a bit busted up. She had a foot issue this week after taking her dog for a long walk. I tried my best to keep the damper on her by writing in "easy pace," but it seems that Heidi only knows one speed—full. She finished drills that were supposed to take 12 minutes in only 7. That was my first glint into Heidi's desire to succeed. She was willing to push as hard as she could to achieve her goal. I realized that it wasn't going to be a lack of effort or work that would hold her back. Her downfall could simply be from her pushing too hard and injuring something. It became very clear that my job was to push her while simultaneously protecting her from going over the edge of her recovery where injury and burnout await. Once you go all the way over the edge, there is no turning back.

SEASON PLANNING

The weekend after Heidi's first week had passed, it was Sunday morning. I worked on my master's thesis Saturday, and afterwards, Jess and I went out to dinner, Thai food at our favorite spot. I ordered the drunken noodles, and Jess chose green curry, her staple dish. I washed my dish down with a draft beer. Jess, a cabernet. Even though I was putting in many hours each week practicing my thesis presentation, which was coming up soon, my mind was now on Heidi and her plight. I told Jess how Heidi's first week went. I also discussed how much planning was involved for her season program, and I felt some nerves in my solar plexus settle. How could I possibly fit in training for all the various capacities that she desired to improve without breaking her? Heidi's list was exhaustive.

Then Jess asked me the big question on Heidi. Why did she want to be a smokejumper so badly? I took a moment to think and said that I didn't ask her and wasn't going to. I told Jess how it felt to talk to Heidi. I described her as having a palpable passion. I could feel her desire through the phone when I spoke with her, thick and electric. She was fully committed. In the spreadsheets, her feedback was humorous, upbeat, and thorough. She wanted to become a smokejumper more than I had wanted to become anything in my life.

Her determination began to rub off on me and compelled me to work as hard as I could to help her. Jess doesn't like it when I talk so much, and I began to sense that she was checking out, so I changed the subject to her classes.

I never did ask Heidi what fueled her extreme desire to become a smokejumper. Sometimes the thought did creep into my mind, though. When it did, I would acknowledge it and then push the question away, telling myself that it was her business alone and not mine to know. I also thought that if she shared her reasons with me, the act of her saying it aloud would decrease the potency of her resolve, somehow jinxing her. She was in charge of her fate. I was simply helping support her.

Heidi wanted to score highly on the PT test, but she also made it very clear that the PT Test that takes place on day one of smokejumper rookie training is "the snowflake on the tip of the iceberg." She wanted me to understand that the PT Test requires a minuscule amount of effort and time compared to the colossal amount of physical work and cognitive demands that are placed on her for the following five-plus weeks beyond day-one testing. Another way to look at this—if you added up all the physical work performed over the entire rookie training duration and compared that to the amount of physical work completed during the PT Test, a snowflake on an iceberg is an accurate depiction. Surpassing the minimum standards was but a small feat compared to the Goliath-tackling task of rookie training in its entirety.

Even though we were a mere half week into working together, Heidi was already physically beyond the BLM minimum standards. However, having experienced rookie training twice already, she had an idea of what she was in for. Passing rookie training is not just about hitting the minimums. You must smash the minimums. It's being able to hit those benchmarks multiple times a day, through week after week of constant physical exertion. Heidi knew that a large part of her success hinged on being able to torch the BLM High Standards any day, any time, in heavy boots, with running in between, and maybe after completing a 12-mile run at elevation through challenging terrain the previous day, and hitting a heavy pack hike and tree climbing prep earlier that morning—all in the middle of a 5-week stint containing similar demands, while learning, memorizing, and executing cognitively demanding parachute jump commands and landing technique.

This is a summary of Heidi's list of secondary training targets beyond the BLM high standards:

- **Running.** Heidi needed to be able to run. A lot. Fast, and far. Sometimes short and fast, too. She listed a range of distances from short sprints to a half marathon. She desired to run a 5k in sub-20 minutes (which equates to about 6:30/mile over 3.1 miles) and a sub-45-minute 10k (7:15/mile for 6.2 miles). These times are not Olympic level by any means, but they are blazing fast compared to the average population of recreational runners. For example, her desired 5k time is in the top 1.79%, meaning she desired to run a faster 5k than 98% of all runners. To keep her competitively fast, over the next few months, Heidi planned to compete twice, hitting a 5k (3.1 miles) and one 10k (6.2 miles), and she had a competitive half marathon trail run (13.1 miles) scheduled in a few weeks. Along with all other training, we were

A taper in sports preparation refers to a period of reduced training load, typically in the weeks leading up to an important competition, with the goal of optimizing an athlete's physical and psychological readiness for peak performance. The purpose of a taper is to balance the athlete's recovery and rest with their need to maintain or improve fitness and performance. During the taper period, the athlete gradually reduces training volume and intensity, allowing the body to recover from the accumulated fatigue of previous training, which allows the body to peak, maximally enhancing their performance potential.

building her weekly running volume progressively with a goal of 40 miles a week before her final taper.

- **Hiking.** Heidi needed to hike frequently with resistances between 60–120 pounds. As mentioned, she only weighed 115 lbs., so the heaviest carries would be at or beyond her bodyweight. Adding difficulty here, smokejumper rookies must ruck their heavy packs and gear at elevation through rugged and steep mountainous terrain. I planned to utilize three different weekly hikes:1) a lighter and longer hike, 2) a medium weight and medium distance hike, and 3) the heavy pack training, usually for 3 flat miles.
- **PT endurance.** Push-ups, pull-ups, and sit-ups. Many days in rookie training contain countless repetitions of these tasks, in boots, with little rest.
- **Core muscle endurance.** Imagine performing hundreds of core-fatiguing movements each day, adding up to thousands of repetitions each week. This was another possible demand of rookie training.
- **Stamina.** Rookie training can last 5–6 weeks, and each week trainees may experience 50+ hours of physical work. Therefore, increasing her hourly, daily, weekly, and monthly work capacity was crucial to Heidi's success.
- **Strength.** Heidi desired a double bodyweight back squat and deadlift (for her, that would be about 250 pounds). The deadlift was much more feasible because Heidi has long femurs that makes squatting more challenging than deadlifting. We also decided that a bodyweight push press would be heavy enough. I was unsure how much emphasis we needed to place on these lifts. The heavy pack test was really the main strength focus. If Heidi could ruck with the 110 lb. pack, and quickly, then she was probably strong enough.
- **Explosive Power.** Explosive power refers to moving one's bodyweight and weighted implements quickly and forcefully, like wielding an axe or sledgehammer, jumping over things, and throwing stuff. Explosive power training is also important to a smokejumper candidate because, in week

three, they enter the parachuting phase of rookie training. Having the ability to produce high amounts of power in training also exposes an athlete to decelerating their bodyweight that transfers nicely to supporting parachute landing practice, which is essentially learning to fall and land in a specific technique to minimize the risk of injury. Heidi desired a bodyweight Power Clean for 5+ reps and a Jerk at 125% of bodyweight. As previously highlighted, Heidi is a small human who will be demanded to do the work of a man 40-60 pounds heavier. Her power levels must be high! In addition, increases in vertical and horizontal jumping ability are desirable. When combined with ideal sprint mechanics, expressing explosive power with one's bodyweight helps create respectable sprint ability. Once sprint mechanics and speed are cultivated, it is a straightforward approach from there to take a good sprinter and teach them to execute agility tasks well. This also helps stabilize the lumbar spine, hips, knees, and ankles.

- **Stability.** To make it through rookie training, Heidi would have to bulletproof her joints and tissues, for which stability plays a huge roll. One of Heidi's main concerns was decreasing or eliminating patellofemoral (knee) pain when descending on long hikes with the heavy packs mentioned above. I had a feeling that simply progressively overloading her heavy pack training, combined with lower body strength training, would serve for Heidi here.
- **Sprint speed.** Heidi informed me that sometimes at rookie training they sprint! She needed to be fast enough to compete with the men. We needed to work her sprint technique and build some volume to inoculate her from the soreness and central nervous system hit that she would take from sprinting without exposure in training.
- **Chronic work capacity.** During rookie training, Heidi would be subjected to many hours of hard labor, testing all the physical capacities and skills listed above, and some that aren't. Therefore, her training must progressively model this demand! I started her at 7 hours of total weekly training time on week 1 and planned to progress her close to more than 20 hours of weekly training in her heaviest training block (5–8 weeks out).
- **Weird things.** As a smokejumper, you might have to climb down from a tree, especially if you get tangled up in one as you parachute into a narrow landing zone on the side of a mountain dense with foliage. I planned to write Heidi specific training tasks and sequences to help prepare her for this unique demand.

Look at that list above. That's a TON of stuff. I had not trained an athlete like this before. This list thoroughly overwhelmed me. Usually, an athlete will tell you that they want to get better at one or two skills or capacities. Sprinters want to be faster and more explosive. Distance runners want to improve their stamina. Throwers want to get stronger and more powerful. Field sport stayed on topic. Rarely would we get off course. We never discussed current events, sports, or politics. It was business only. And the business was hard training.

Me: "Find a 5RM but leave a few reps 'in the tank,' i.e. don't get a true max. Take at least 90" between your heaviest final sets"

Heidi: "45#, 65#, 95# as 5rm, 4:45 w/ 90" rest between each. I need 2.5, 5, and 15 weights and weight rack, I'll go to mikes after the month in Santa Barbara"

Me: "Sounds good. How was the heels elevated addition to the front squats?"

Heidi: "Felt good!"

Me: "Great. I'll keep using this for a while."

Heidi: "Went up to 5 reps at 105"

She didn't ask about my personal life, and I didn't pry into hers. The only time I would ask such questions was if her personal life began to go against the grain of her training goals. So far, she was on course and very consistent. She showed up each week to training with the right attitude to conquer her quest. However, her foot was still bothersome. She wrote in the spreadsheets that the pain was gone and her foot was feeling numb. While this seemed like an improvement to her, I knew that numbness was ominous.

MONDAY, NOVEMBER 14, 2016 (22 WEEKS OUT)

After three and a half weeks of training, at Heidi's request, I added road biking and mountain biking into Heidi's weekly conditioning regimen to accompany her swimming. We used the road bike for recovery rides, and she used the mountain bike on hilly and challenging terrain to perform unstructured intervals. Her feedback was always succinct and cutely funny. She'd tell me how tough the mountain bike ride was and usually provided the trail's name. On a light pack hike one day, this was her feedback, "2hr15min Fun hike at Del Rosa! Hiked my hotshot hikes: meatball, dead air, the one, all the bonuses and the parallel to the one. Not sure on distance forgot my gps watch :/ about 15–20 lbs." To this day, I have no idea what those hikes are, how steep, or the terrain type. All that mattered to me was hearing that she enjoyed the hike, carried weight on it, experienced some elevation gain/loss, and went for about two hours. Her feedback was always matter of fact. It seemed that she thought I knew all the trail names, where they were, how challenging, and good completion times for each. I don't think that Heidi knew how much I didn't know about some of the topics that she spoke about during our conversations. She would speak so quickly, and we had so much to cover, that I didn't really have time to ask her to elaborate on some of the smaller details.

That week the heavy pack training was 40 pounds, and Heidi practiced hiking in boots. Her feedback can be hysterical. "My crazy woman walk course is quite interesting but it works :) I felt good and was able to keep my pace and entertain the town of forest falls at the same time :)." She is referring to her athletes want to improve their ability to change direction and stop on a dime. Heidi was a different animal entirely. She made it seem like she would wash out this year if we didn't train every item on the list, and she made it clear to me that we needed to maximize many of the tasks. Due to my lack of experience in smokejumper preparation, I didn't know how to prioritize which capacities we needed to spend more time on and which we could put on the back burner, so I went for an approach of shooting to steadily take them all down over the next six months. It was a high-risk, high-reward approach. Heidi was willing to risk it all.

While programming out my theoretical training blocks and progressions for Heidi over the upcoming six months, I kept in my mind the power of chronic adaptations. She didn't need to max every day. She didn't need to reach her physical peak by the end of next week, either. I decided to play the long game. Throughout the upcoming six months, her body would adapt to similar and progressive stimuli while we steadily added training intensity and volume, all with the goal of consistently demanding a series of small physiological adaptations. Throughout this time, each small adaptation would compound to facilitate chronic changes in muscle tissue endurance and strength; significant changes to skeletal bone mineral density, ligament and tendon thickness, endocrine responses, metabolic adaptations; and fascial remodeling to match and support her movement patterns.

Intensity refers to the relative difficulty of a task. For example, in strength training, coaches often use percentages of an athlete's heaviest lift, called percentage-based training. Percentage-based training is common with barbell tasks like squatting, deadlifting, pressing, and Olympic Weightlifting. Rate of Perceived Exertion, abbreviated as RPE, is also used. This is a rating scale, usually between 1–10, where 1 is easy and 10 is the most challenging that you can imagine. I often use RPE for prescribing running and hiking workouts. If I suggested a 5-mile run at an RPE of 6.0, that means run five miles at a pace that feels like a 6 out of 10 in difficulty.

There really is no way to train all capacities simultaneously to any degree of proficiency while keeping the athlete alive to tell the tale, so I utilized programming structural knowledge gleaned through my experience at U of I when I worked under Mike and Tonja, which was rehashed over the past few years in my master's program. To help me organize everything into a format that made sense, I sat at my kitchen table with an oversized piece of paper and a high quality #2 drafting pencil and sketched out some hypothetical training blocks.

I thought about the preseason planning at U of I with Mike, sitting down in front of the whiteboard to plan the training season, backwards. The six-month training duration from now until mid-April when Heidi left for rookie training would be my macrocycle, the largest training block. Within this, I designated

4-week blocks as mesocycles. Within each of those 4-week blocks, I set four microcycles, each a single week in duration. My plan was to use a wave cycle of loading for most of Heidi's training, including her PT tasks (pull-ups, push-ups, and sit-ups), running, and strength training. I learned how to do this after following Pavel's programming lessons from his books. For progressing the pack training, I planned to rely on a linear loading cycle, meaning that we would add weight every week. This idea came from a training document provided to Heidi by Matt Bowers. The main principle of the document suggested that a linear progression allowed connective tissue and bone enough time to adapt over months of loading. I had a feeling that we could not add weight indefinitely, but I wanted to see how far I could take her with this plan. Even the best athletes cannot improve continuously in one linear climb. Progress is gained through peaks and valleys which, if everything goes well enough, trend upwards.

In training design, many coaches break up training blocks into microcycles, mesocycles, and macrocycles. Microcycles are the shortest, usually a week. Mesocycles are longer and consist of 3–8 microcycles lasting 1–2 months. Mesocycles are the largest and comprise several mesocycles, lasting 3–12 months.

In classic periodization models, each microcycle within a mesocycle contains a specific amount of volume, and each block is different than the previous. The mesocycle structure I utilized for Heidi increased the volume each week for four weeks, and then the beginning of the next block served as a deload where the volume was decreased to allow for recovery before building more volume in the new mesocycle.

On paper, Heidi's program was filling out nicely. However, I had no idea how this would all work out. When you plan ahead, you are guessing at how the athlete will progress. Sometimes they grow in quick upward spurts. Other times, they plateau. Occasionally, a big life event occurs and the whole plan must be scrapped or rewritten. I hoped that my estimates for her capabilities and speed of progression were accurate. Her success depended on it.

The heavy pack test was a specific training stimulus at the top of Heidi's list. On day one of rookie training during Heidi's second year and second attempt, she hoisted the 110 lb. pack onto her back and walked the three flat miles. She finished over the time cap, and they washed her immediately. On day one. Not fit for duty. To say the heavy pack training would be a mainstay in our weekly training is an understatement. In my mind, the heavy pack training was the steak, and everything else was carrots.

In the world of wildland fire, pack tests are common. A pack test is carrying a "pack" for distance and time. A pack is a large bag filled with weight and worn on the back like a backpack. Often, athletes will purchase a ruck sack, which is a specific backpack created to allow the user to load up the pack with resistance. Rucksacks often have both shoulder straps like a backpack and a hip strap like a camping or hiking pack. For training purposes, Heidi had a pack that she could load with over a hundred pounds. We needed to utilize every square inch of this pack by the time she left for rookie training!

> Wave cycles utilize progressive loading of training volume over a mesocycle. Imagine a month of training where the first week is easy, the second week is a little tougher, the third tougher still, and the fourth is toughest. Four-week mesocycle complete! The next 4-week mesocycle may contain a little more volume in each week, culminating in week 8 with the highest volume yet, higher than week 4s peak.

Pack tests are specific to the demands of the job. Smokejumpers often parachute with over 90 pounds of gear and supplies and must hike to the fire line and then back out again with the gear, minus consumed food and water. For the smokejumper selection process, the pack test is 110 pounds carried for three miles in under 65 minutes on a flat course. Heidi warned me about this test. She only weighed 115 pounds when we began working together (her bodyweight was a separate training issue because there is a minimum body-weight for safety reasons while parachuting), so that pack test load was almost her bodyweight!

Years later, Heidi wrote:

"I would do this test on the flat part of Valley of the Falls drive where it comes off HWY 38 and turns around at the bridge... I'm sure people thought I was crazy (ha, ha!) or just confused. Once I did a lap by Sierra's house and later she told me she saw this poor woman with a hunch back struggling in the rain and I said 'that was me!'"

To help her prepare for this grueling test, I looked up some articles outlining training strategies for improving pack test performance. The most useful article suggested a linear periodization to build up bone and connective tissue strength while allowing the aerobic system to adapt. Bones and connective tissue take months at minimum to garner usable adaptations, so that's the route I picked for her. We started out with just 30 pounds the first week and kept the distance to three miles. From here out, I planned for Heidi to complete a heavy pack training session every single week. My plan was to increase load on this task by 5–10 pounds every week until it got heavy for her. At that point, I had another plan.

Her foot pain was present during pack training as well, but she plugged along, using what she calls her "shuffle-run technique," which is faster than a walk and slower than a jog. For the first few weeks, every time I wrote her pack training, in the back of my mind, I was concerned that this would be the thing that would break her during our preparation. It was the heaviest and consistently one of the longer duration training pieces each week. Working up to a fast near-body-weight carry is no joke!

Heidi's living arrangement added difficulty to her training. She was living in Forest Falls, California, a little mountain town nestled halfway up the west side of the San Bernardino Mountains. Her house was more than a mile above sea level, about 5,800 feet, which was perfect for high altitude training. She had plenty of hikes near her, including San Gorgonio, San Bernardino, and a few other 10,000–11,500-foot peaks, the trailheads all within walking distance of her home. In a month or two, it would begin to snow in Forest Falls, and much of that would stick around until March or April.

Perhaps the craziest part of this entire coach/athlete relationship was the fact that Heidi was going to tackle all this training on her own. My job was less coach and more programmer, meaning that I would write into our shared spreadsheet what she should do, and she'd do it. If I had seen her in person a few days a week, I might have gotten a better idea of how she moved, what she needed, and how to progress each task based on what I saw with my own eyes. However, logistically this wouldn't work. Heidi had to perform the work on her own, and we had to develop systems of communication through text and the spreadsheets, and sometimes phone calls, to ensure that we were on the same page. Any miscommunications could prove catastrophic.

SUNDAY, OCTOBER 30, 2016 (25 WEEKS OUT)

Heidi's first full week of training came and went. I was relieved that we made it through without any new nagging residual issues popping up from the fire season. Heidi realized that she was more out of shape than she thought! I kept the training light. She completed a decent initial volume of push-ups, pull-ups, sit-ups, bodyweight squats and lunges, and core work. Since Heidi had CrossFit experience and mentioned that she wanted to increase her strength and power, I also wrote in barbell movements like deadlifts, front squats, and power cleans. Kettlebell swings were part of her first training block, too, and once again, I utilized many of Pavel's principles to design her kettlebell training progressions.

Her foot continued to give her trouble that week, so she could not run yet. Running is a huge part of the rookie training, so I was keen to help her heal this foot issue as quickly and completely as we could, given our short and intense training timeline. Instead of running, we initially relied on swimming to improve her aerobic capacity, and I also had her perform fast walking. Since Heidi lived more than a mile above sea level in Forest Falls, California, walking fast at that altitude proved effective to enhance her conditioning while we rehabbed her foot. I was concerned that this foot issue would become her "Achilles heel."

Despite her foot, Heidi's mindset was strong. She was warming up quickly to me as her coach. One and a half weeks of training had passed, and we were building rapport. She was getting to know my coaching and programming style, and I was getting to know her better as an athlete and a person. Despite the drab cliché of a spreadsheet, I found myself enjoying our interactions through rows and columns of text conversations within the programming. She was not afraid to be herself, making little jokes and writing in noises and creating different emojis. I could immediately feel her emotion through her feedback. After a 1-hour hike, she wrote, "3.43 miles Momyer Creek Trail in FF. No weight, no fire boots. Hiked right after strength, had an apple, was a lil tired but felt good on my mad woman hike! Glutes burned but it was great! Hammies a lil tight but I'll stretch tonight."

It was difficult to focus on programming for Heidi that week because the Chicago Cubs were playing the Cleveland Indians for the 2016 baseball World Series. For those who aren't baseball fans, the last Cubs' World Series Title was 108 years before, the longest-ever World Series drought. Although Jess and I are both from Chicago, I'm a Sox fan and Jess loves the Cubbies. Over the years, we had gone to a few Sox vs. Cubs games dressed in our respective team's jerseys, and her damn Cubs bested my Sox every single time, which is rough for me because Jess is a great shit-talker and takes pride in prodding me with her dry wit. But tonight, during game 7, I was a Cubs fan. In this series, the Cubs were down 3 games to 1 and were still alive after winning the last two games. With the series tied at three games, a win for the Cubs would prove an amazing comeback, extremely rare in the world of sport, especially with the world title on the line.

Jess's grandmother, a life-long, die-hard Cubs fan, who had never seen them win the World Series, had passed away earlier that year, and Jess was a crumpled pile in the living room, her limbs limp, eyes red with tears of frustration as the Indians steadily clobbered their way back to a 6–6 score by the 9th inning, just in time for a rain delay. The suspense was immense! In extra innings, through the rain, after more than four and a half hours, with an 8–7 lead in the bottom of the 10th inning, the Cubs earned a final strikeout, winning the game and the World Series Title. Jess and I hugged and kissed, and she cried some more.

After the excitement of the game subsided, I realized that Heidi was working towards a comeback story of her own, one that stretched through two failed rookie training attempts over two years. It was unheard of to attempt a third run at rookie training. She said this would be her final attempt. We had to get it right.

SUNDAY, NOVEMBER 6, 2016 (23 WEEKS OUT)

Every Sunday morning, often after hitting the downtown bars hard the night before with old college friends who still lived in the area, I would sit down at my oversized kitchen table with my planning documents, computer, and

18x24-inch sketch pad for a few hours, and I would craft Heidi's upcoming week of training. It felt very similar to creating art. For most of my life up to these recent years that I spent coaching, I was an artist, a potter, and sculptor. My planning process for Heidi felt like a nice blend between art and science. I relied on everything I knew from the practical world of strength and conditioning and blended in my own intuition, and it felt that I was creating a giant work of art. My palate was a combination of track and field principles from working with Mike and Tonja to improve her running and hiking; strength training knowledge gleaned from Pavel's books to improve her strength, power, and PT score; and CrossFit to improve her work capacity.

Heidi had many years of CrossFit experience, so she knew how to push herself in a metabolic conditioning session (metcon), and I was hoping that her volume tolerance was high enough for me to push her on the running and hiking, eventually, after her foot healed. That was still bothering her. Heidi's strength was sound for a woman her size, and her volume tolerance for PT tasks like strict pull-ups, push-ups, sit-ups, and other bodyweight and lightly loaded tasks was excellent. She had the makings of a "physical specimen," a freak. All we had to do was put the pieces together over the remaining five months and hope that she stayed in one piece.

In addition to Heidi's massive list of training considerations and targets, Heidi weighed about 115 pounds at the end of her last fire season. This was problematic for smokejumping because the minimum bodyweight was 120 pounds. Gaining weight while increasing running and weighted hiking volume was an additional challenge. Add in Heidi's desire to break her personal best marks in the PT Test (pull-ups, push-ups, sit-ups, and the 1.5-mile run), which are all bodyweight tasks, meaning that the records are more easily broken at a lighter bodyweight, and now the situation became even more challenging. Heidi demanded excellence of herself, and in turn, this was mirrored back to me to help her attain her lofty goals.

> A metcon, in the CrossFit world, is shorthand for metabolic conditioning, which is a term used to describe a training strategy that relies on combining strength training, gymnastics, and cardiovascular training methods together into one intense and (usually) short training session. Metcons are a type of HIT (High Intensity Training) and HIIT (High Intensity Interval Training).

Even though she might be faster and be able to perform better on the PT test at a lighter weight, we had to get her bodyweight up to meet the minimum standard. I suggested that she begin to eat a little more food so that she gained the weight slowly. Since we had just over five months remaining, all she had to do was gain about one pound each month. When bodyweight is put on slowly and while undergoing a progressive strength training program, there is an increased probability that most of the weight gained is muscle mass. It would do Heidi no good at all to gain five pounds of body fat. It would weigh her down on every task. However, if we could increase her muscle mass by five pounds, or more, all that muscle would provide more strength for her body-weight tasks, and more power in her legs for the heavy pack test and carrying her pack up the jump tower for multiple reps a day. Since she had to gain the weight, might as well make the weight work optimally for her.

I had some nutritional experience, but not much. I suggested a simple approach. Eat a little more food each day by increasing her fullness at dinner-time. The rest of her meals she could keep the same. To clean up her diet further, I suggested she rely on eat lean meats, plenty of starchy carbohydrates like potatoes and rice, lots of fruit, and healthy fats from avocados and nuts. I didn't need to tell her to lay off alcohol and eating out at restaurants where the nutritional content was not under her control. She was proving herself dedicated in the gym, and I assumed that she would also be diligent with her food intake.

Volume tolerance is an athlete's ability to recover from specific volumes of training stress. Training volume is calculated by multiplying the number of total repetitions completed by the resistance. Here are three simple examples of how to calculate for three different training stimuli:

- 30 barbell back squats at 100 pounds = 30 x 100 = 3,000 pounds (back squat volume)
- 3 days in one week with pull-ups, total reps = 250 (pull-up volume)
- 120 miles of running completed in one month (month volume)

You can track pounds lifted, miles run and hiked, repetitions completed, and training duration in minutes or hours. Once volume is calculated, you can compare that with your athlete's recovery data while undergoing that volume to decide how much to push them next time.

Each week, I delivered Heidi's training through Google spreadsheets, which was a new delivery method for me. On one of the tabs, I wrote up her training for the week. On another tab, I created a weekly tracking feature where I could compare her training volumes from week to week for each important task. I also used the planning tab to shape her season plan, building in peak weeks and deload weeks in attempt to optimize her adaptations.

A deload is a lighter volume and/or intensity stretch of time that allows the athlete to recover and prepare for the next increase in training volume and/or intensity. A single deload week is common during heavy training, and multiple consecutive deload weeks can be useful in the off-season to stimulate full recovery of the athlete's bodily systems.

Heidi and I got to know each other well through the spreadsheets. There were sometimes five or six different exchanges back and forth on a single line featuring one specific aspect of her training for that week. Most of the time we positive affirmations mantra that she says out loud while hiking around her little mountain town. Imagine a tiny muscley-hamster Heidi hiking around your neighborhood with a big pack on her back, loudly talking to herself.

At the beginning of this trek towards rookie training, I suggested that Heidi create and recite personal mantras while training. This is what she was yelling on her "crazy woman walk course" through her town. She began to practice this habit on long hikes, long runs, and particularly difficult PT training sessions to help her get through the session with a strong mind. I urged her to use powerful language and to remind herself after each tough training session that she was growing stronger and stronger.

Belief in the power of a mantra is extremely important. Not only must Heidi believe in the words that she speaks, but she should also believe in the practice itself. Layering in this belief takes thousands of reps and hundreds of miles of effort, and once at rookie training, when the going gets tough, the mantras would hopefully help her through the darkness. After practicing repetitions of her mantras through increasingly tougher training sessions, we ingrained this habit. She was able to reason with herself that she'd made it through everything up to this point, and that she'd make it through this, too. This type of mental strategy helped keep Heidi at the optimal level of arousal. If she felt her energy or mindset slipping downward, she could pick herself back up by reciting her mantra.

Meanwhile, my schedule was packed. I woke up at 5:40 a.m. (on Tuesdays, I coached the 5:00 a.m. class and woke up at 4:20 a.m. to open the gym at 4:50 a.m.), threw on my gym coaching clothes, brushed my teeth, and then I went straight to work from 6 to 10 in the morning. After that shift, I'd hit my own training until noon, come home for lunch, spend time with Jess if she wasn't busy with her own studies, maybe swim some laps in the apartment pool which was always empty, practice a run-through or two of my master's thesis presentation, then back to work from 4 p.m. until closing around 8 p.m. Next, home for dinner with Jess, and then we'd sit down and together enjoy some *Goliath* (Billy Bob Thornton at his best) or *Walking Dead*, and then back to bed. Rinse and repeat. On the weekends, I'd sleep in until 9 or 10 a.m. to catch up on my sleep debt from the previous week.

Jessica and I were in school for different things. She was working on a degree in Clinical Lab Science (CLS). We had been living in Redlands for just over four years, and Jessica wanted out. She was sick of the fact that I.E. Redlands was a small town and seemed to stifle her growth. I think she knew it from the moment we arrived on the day she overheated in her little Cavalier.

Three years before this, she had spied a route out of Redlands and began to pursue it. She began working at a research lab through Loma Linda University, a small private school in the next town. She worked under Dr. Lee Berk and volunteered to help him run his lab where they studied the effects of dark chocolate on the brain and other interesting research on human performance. Dr. Berk was her "in" at this university. She loved working with Dr.

Berk. Over the next year, she completed her prerequisites and was accepted into Loma Linda's clinical lab science bachelor's degree program (she already had her bachelor's degree in biology from the University of Illinois in Champaign-Urbana, where we met. This degree would be her second). And once she got her degree, she planned to get a job working for the highest paying healthcare company in the state of California, Kaiser Permanente, and she wanted to move to a bigger city in California. We were eyeing San Diego and San Francisco. Jess was well on her way to actualizing this dream for us. She was slated to graduate the next year, in July of 2017.

It was time for my thesis defense presentation in Cedar City, Utah! I drove up from Redlands to Cedar City the night before my presentation. During the drive, I practiced my presentation and went over my slides in my head. The driving was slow once I got past the Arizona-Utah border. The other drivers and I were hit with an unexpected snowstorm. I had to slow down to about 25 miles an hour for the last few hours of the drive due to low visibility, wind, and a bit of ice on the road. The adrenaline from the rough driving conditions mixed with my excitement about my thesis defense, and by the end of the trip, I was wide awake. I got into town late and missed dinner. Cedar City is one of those small towns that closes at 9 p.m. I checked into my hotel and spent most of the night tossing and turning.

The next morning, I woke up a few hours early to make sure that everything for my presentation was in order. I had been working on this thesis for the past two years. While getting dressed, in a panic, I realized that I had forgotten my button-down shirt for the presentation at home! My heart began to race as adrenaline surged, and I began to sweat as I went through a freak out. I calmed down enough to realize that I had just enough time to go find a shirt. I found a clothing store and bought a light purple button-down shirt that fit well enough, then drove over to the classroom for my defense.

I had been through my material a hundred times, and I'd had the honor of practicing this presentation in front of the physical therapy faculty at Loma Linda University a few times. Today, I presented my thesis on collegiate female rugby athletes to Dr. Thomas, my thesis chair, and the rest of the Southern Utah University master's program staff, including Joan, the secretary for the department. She had been working there for more than forty years and watched most of the presentations during her tenure.

I chose to study the relationship between speed, power, and strength in collegiate female rugby athletes. On the side a few nights a week for the past few years, I was the strength coach for a team of female rugby players from the University of California Riverside, a neighboring city. When deciding what to study for my thesis, the rugby team was a no-brainer, and the process was straightforward and enjoyable.

It took me about 30 minutes to present, and then I defended my research for another 30 minutes, answering questions posed by the staff, Dr. Thomas, and Joan. For the first time in my life, I felt good presenting. In the past,

I would get anxious and lose my composure, forgetting important details, stumbling when asked questions. This time around, through sheer repetition of practice and a thorough understanding of my research, I nailed it. I felt present and poised for the entire presentation and defense. Afterwards, Joan pulled me aside to congratulate me on one of the best thesis defenses that she had ever seen. I was so relieved! I felt amazing. However, all that truly mattered was whether my knowledge and experience translated to real-world success for Heidi and other athletes like her.

Afterwards, I wanted to celebrate, but I didn't really know anyone, so I took myself out for a late lunch. I went to a barbecue place in the middle of town. I had been there the previous year for some on-campus classes, so I knew the small town well enough. The meal was good, and I washed it down with a low alcohol percentage brown ale brewed within the state of Utah. Then I hit the road back home, driving late into the night. I drove fast and kept the music loud, singing along and dancing a bit in the driver's seat. I had done it! My defense was over!!

On the drive home, I called Jess and told her how it went. I think she was more relieved than I was. In my excitement, I also called Heidi. She congratulated me and then we discussed how her training was going. One of the things that I had noticed and enjoyed about Heidi was her willingness to try something new. I found this remarkable, and I told her so. She just laughed it off and said she completely put her trust in me and found the novelty of our coaching relationship exciting and simple. All she had to do was show up and do what was written. At least that's how she felt. I knew it ran deeper than that. Much deeper. In fact, I believe that it ran all the way to the core of who she was. She already had good habits to support her training. She ate well, kept a regular sleeping schedule, and maintained healthy relationships in her life. While these things may seem trivial, like they don't connect with her training, I strongly believe they do matter. A lot. If one's personal relationships are problematic, they don't sleep well. They are unsettled during the day. Their recovery suffers. Poor eating habits also affect recovery and performance. Poor sleep has detrimental effects on everything, including training, appetite, recovery, and even how we interact with others.

Training with a coach like me was a very new experience for Heidi. Someone stepping in and guiding every aspect of what she should do for training each week was a huge change of pace from the fly-by-the-seat-of-her-pants unstructured training that she was used to. She would try new hikes that she hadn't trekked before. Sometimes they would not fit what she was looking for. Her feedback in the spreadsheets was entertaining to me as she described these mini failures, just as long as she didn't get injured along the way. She always learned from her experiences, and I think that was one of her greatest strengths—her curiosity and fearlessness when trying out a new route, both real and hypothetical.

At long last, after fast walking, mountain biking, and swimming for the past month, Heidi began running again. I chose to reintroduce her to running using intervals of walk, then jog, followed by a short run.

Training: Running = 30 mins: 5 rounds – 2 min. walk, 3 min. easy jog, 1 min. medium speed run!

Heidi's feedback: "Fun!! Felt amazing! Free! Ran on Aliso canyon trail in the Los padres NF. 2.62 miles"

These sequences seemed to be enough stress to improve her running while not aggravating her foot injury. Her foot seemed to be healing, slowly. In her feedback, Heidi wrote that her foot was not in pain, but was just *numb*. That word again. This wasn't the first time her foot had felt numb. To her, numb was an improvement because her pain was gone. However, I cautioned her that numb wasn't necessarily a good thing and to continue paying attention to it. This really worried me. I hoped that her foot would hold up through the training. For her to be successful, I believed that we had to push her running and hiking volume quite a bit further than her current capabilities.

Every couple of weeks, Heidi and I would hop on a phone call to touch base. While weekly Monday and Friday text check-ins were helpful, I was constantly monitoring her results through the spreadsheet a few days each week to ensure that I was up to speed on her progress. However, phone calls were really the best way for us to catch up in a clear, detailed, and time efficient manner. It was on one of these calls that Heidi let me know another detail about the Boise Smokejumper Base.

Skipping the small talk and jumping right into the meat of things, matter-of-factly Heidi told me that, in her opinion, rookieing out of Boise was the toughest route to become a smokejumper. She had put Boise on a pedestal and wanted to earn a spot amongst the top wildland firefighters in the country. She could have chosen a different base to rookie out of and transferred into Boise, like so many had done before. Instead, she had sought the toughest challenge that she could find. This desire to test and prove oneself against the greatest possible challenge is what designates her as unique and elite.

While coaching Heidi in 2016 and 2017, I didn't know her backstory. I didn't have the bandwidth in my life to ask such questions. I was a coach, so I coached. Knowing or not knowing her backstory had no bearing on how I trained her. Seven years later, I finally asked her how she got into fire. She writes: "I did an internship with the USFS when I was in college and learned about Del Rosa hotshots ... I continued college to get my masters and started working at Esri in Redlands. Great job! But wanted something more physically challenging ... 3 years after working at Esri I contacted Del Rosa and asked what I needed to do to become a hotshot and so I started training then. 2–3 times a day on my own to meet the minimum fitness requirements at that time and be able to keep up on hikes. So, once they saw I could keep up on hikes I applied and got picked up. That was 7 years after the initial meeting with the hotshot crew."

After spending a few years on the notorious Del Rosa Hotshots, Heidi began applying to smokejumper bases. Subsequent conversations revealed some old psychological wounds that she was holding onto. Each week in her feedback, she remembered another part of the previous year's rookie training challenges and would ask me to add the antidote to it into her training. After a few of these requests, I realized that she needed some mindset drills to help her overcome past failures to quell fears and unblock her potential. In extreme situations, an athlete is only as strong as their weakest aspect of their mindset. I believed if Heidi brought these fears with her into rookie training, they would sap her energy and confidence and ultimately bring about her demise in this third and final attempt.

TUESDAY, NOVEMBER 29, 2016 (20 WEEKS OUT)

Heidi completed her first partial PT test. She hit 16 strict pull-ups, 66 push-ups, and 100 sit-ups. These numbers are already well beyond the Boise minimum standards! I was happy. That week Heidi was home for Thanksgiving and only trained for a few days. I should have written her a heavy deload week and given her time off to spend with her family, but I didn't. She trained through this week, which was a mistake on my part. I did not factor in the holiday. Big mistake.

The initial sign of a setback arrived Monday and Tuesday of the next week. On Monday, Heidi mentioned "falling off the motivational boat for a bit," and Tuesday, "the kb soured a mental breakdown." I immediately felt an ache begin to develop in my gut, and throughout the week, it panged louder. I had pushed her for too many weeks in a row and through the Thanksgiving holiday week without a break. Heidi's negative feedback was new, and I paid close attention. It felt like we were beginning to overreach, meaning that her physical workload had become greater than her ability to recover. This saps the body and mind of motivation, and eventually causes tiny physical issues that can grow into larger problems. I had been wondering when she would begin to feel this way. We were pushing hard consistently. I had her training six days a week for 2–3 hours a day.

A day later, on Wednesday, for her heavy pack training (which was now at 51 pounds), Heidi wrote in the spreadsheets that she "felt tired physically and mentally." This was my third and final sign that she needed to deload, and soon. I noted in her sheets that we would drop the volume a bit the following week to allow her body to recover.

As a track athlete, I remember experiencing overreaching, although at the time, I just felt shitty all-around. I couldn't sleep well. My usually humongous appetite fizzled. My relationships felt overwhelming; I fell behind on my classwork and was unable to meet expectations everywhere. This usually hit me from the middle to end of a long and arduous track and field season.

The stress from training is intimately connected to our physiology, along with a host of "other" factors and can be lumped into categories like nutrition, sleep, and psychological stress from work, family, friends, commuting, and other situations. When any of these areas are out of balance, training can take a hit, causing a tough training week.

Stress also combines with other factors from mid-terms, big projects, and relationship issues. As an athlete, I thought that I was uniquely weak, unable to mentally hack it as well as my colleagues at times. When coaching at U of I, I realized the stress effects I had experienced were not unique to me and that every athlete on the team was challenged by psychological stressors which affected their performance to some extent, especially later in the season when physical stress from practice was close to maximum and the weekly competition travel schedule seemingly endless, all compounded by the expectations to produce apex competitive performances every weekend.

Each of those stressors influences an individual athlete's physiology. It does not matter where the stress originates. Too much of any one stressor or an overload of a combination of stressors can cause injury, burnout, or both. I saw this trend developing in Heidi and knew we had to back off immediately.

I had two choices here—to ask Heidi why she was faltering, or to simply change her training volume without mentally probing. I chose the latter, because Heidi was the type of athlete that, when asked why she's not performing up to a standard (set by me, her, or elsewhere), would break herself to meet the standard. It was too early in the season for her to push dangerously close to her physiological edge, so I went with the latter solution and changed training volume without asking her and hoped that was the best decision.

Here are some of my main signs that an athlete is having a tough week of training and may need a few rest days or a deload week:

- **Frustration.** The athlete's feedback shows psychological frustration or negativity with how they are performing, whether their performances are actually bad or not. Sometimes athletes are performing below expectations through training and life circumstances, and if they perceive this negatively or become frustrated with themselves or me, I must set them straight. If they are doing well and aren't seeing things clearly, then I can teach them what I see to help quell their concerns. If they actually are underperforming, that's another issue.
- **Performance.** The athlete is performing below what is expected of them at the current moment.
- **Recovery.** If an athlete begins to feel their recovery is slowing down between training sessions, this is a sure sign of an imbalance of stressors. One main factor is the speed of healing one's skin. If cuts and scrapes take longer to heal, this is a sign that the body's recovery resources are strained.
- **Soreness.** Extra tissue soreness that takes longer than usual to heal.

- **Desire to train.** Here is a difference between soreness, fatigue, and desire to train. They are separate sensations. An athlete can wake up feeling sore, fatigued, and may still have a strong desire to train. Conversely, they can wake up feeling fresh and have a low desire to train. Each of these scenarios are useful for the coach to know.
- **Sleep.** Their sleep patterns change. This could be a desire to sleep much more, or much less. More sleep may suggest their body is overstressed and craving more sleep to help balance their stress equation. This may be ok as long as performance holds up. Less sleep may suggest their anxiety is increasing, keeping them from falling asleep, staying asleep, or causing them to wake up earlier than they should.
- **Appetite.** Any changes in appetite could signify an imbalance of stress. Athletes tend to under eat when overstressed.
- **Stool.** There is a stool consistency guide called the Bristol Stool Chart. Stools are classified from 1–7, in which lower scores are firmer (1-class stools signify constipation) to looser (7-class stools signify diarrhea). Most of the time, when an athlete is stressed beyond an optimal level, stools will move towards the higher end of the range. Optimal stool consistency is right in the middle of the gradient, classified as a 3 or a 4.

These signs suggest that an athlete is overreaching and headed towards overtraining. There are two main choices for a coach when an athlete begins to show an imbalance of stressors. One, we can make training easier to give the athlete's recovery system a chance to catch up; or two, we can help guide the athlete to improve their recovery. Improving recovery could entail teaching an athlete how to change their habits to improve sleep quantity or quality or to clean up their nutrition. Maybe they aren't eating enough and need more food to help them recover, or maybe they have some bad relationships in their life that they must learn to accept or discard. When an athlete like Heidi has an all-encompassing athletic goal, these conversations must take place. A coach who fails to address these realities leaves room for failure.

Overtraining syndrome occurs when an athlete's training stressors outweigh their recovery ability and practices. Over a few weeks to months, this uneven relationship can cause many unwanted outcomes. Overreaching is a phase along the continuum between healthy adaptation to training and overtraining:

[untrained]<>[detrained]<> **[optimal zone]** <>[overreaching]<>[overtraining]<>[injury/burnout]

With Heidi, I knew that she was optimizing her nutrition, sleep, and she kept her social life simple enough that stress arising from issues with other people was not a problem, so if she displayed any of the above signs of stress imbalance, then I assumed that it was almost certainly training related.

For this week, I went back into her training on Wednesday night and dialed back her volume for the rest of the week. I realized this made it very difficult to project my programming for her more than a few weeks ahead. In an ideal world, I would steadily progress her every week until rookie training, and she would respond wonderfully to everything that I gave her. However, this is not how the world works. No one responds favorably to physical training every single day, week, and month, especially a seasoned wildland firefighter with years of experience like Heidi.

With our sights on the start of rookie training, if we were conservative, I would have been able to estimate what volume she could handle each week and month as we progressed. This would have been the safest approach, but it also would yield a lower level of final performance. In other words, the degree of progress sloping up towards day one would be less steep if we took a conservative approach. However, that could leave untapped gains that we could have garnered if we pushed harder. What if those untapped gains were the thing that could make the difference between Heidi passing or washing? She had failed twice already. This was her final attempt. We both felt that pressure.

How hard to push? We couldn't do too much training. She would go into rookie training too brittle, and she'd break. Not too little training either, or she'd go in flat and then begin to break down mentally because she'd be physically under prepared. This had happened in the past at McCall. So, we shot at the upper middle of those extremes. I pushed her as hard as I could without breaking her. The problem with pushing as hard as possible is that you don't know where the edge is. It's awfully fun to be on the edge. Imagine sitting on the edge of a cliff with a thousand-foot drop below, swinging your legs like a kid on a swing. It's exhilarating! As an athlete, you feel kind of like this when pushing very hard in training. The edge is also dangerous. You can fall off and die. In training, people don't often die, but they can get seriously injured or burned out. Understand that once you push an athlete over the edge, they break. And the comeback process may not be salvaged in days or weeks, but instead may take months or years. We didn't have the luxury of time to rehab Heidi if she broke. We had to get it right the first go-around.

In early December, coincidentally it seems, I began to write mental training drills directly into Heidi's spreadsheets. And just in time, too. I hoped that adding this element would help accelerate her up to the next level of physical and psychological growth. To begin our journey towards improved mindset and mental control over her physiology, we kept it very simple—10 minutes of mindfulness each day. I also gave her some homework and suggested that she read a book called *Full Catastrophe Living*, by Jon Kabat-Zinn, and suggested she try a drill from that book called the "raisin meditation" for a few minutes each day when she ate.

Kabat-Zinn's "raisin meditation" is a drill in mindfulness. Mindfulness is to practice consciousness within the present moment. It requires noticing what is happening around and within you, without judgment. To apply this concept to a raisin, you take a single raisin and place it on the table in front of you. Spend a few moments appreciating it's textures, colors, how the light hits the many ridges and swirls in its skin. Then you pick up the raisin and hold it, feeling its weight and texture. Squeeze it between your fingertips to sense the pressure the little fruit pushes back against the world with. Smell the raisin, noticing its unique and surprisingly varied and rich aroma. Then think about eating it: what the raisin would taste like, what it would feel like on your tongue, what the raisin would feel like as you bite it in half with your front teeth and mash it between your molars. Then you take an actual bite and notice how it actually feels to bite into and chew the raisin. What flavors do you notice? How much saliva have you produced? How wonderful was that single raisin? Congratulations! You just spend a minute or two in the present moment. You weren't living in the past, replaying some highlight or blooper reel, and you weren't living in the future, either, concerned about your to-do list. You were in the here and now. And how beautiful it is! This was Heidi's first lesson in mindfulness. She felt that this eating meditation was fun.

MONDAY, DECEMBER 12, 2016 (18 WEEKS OUT)

Jessica and I snuck home for Christmas that week. We only spent a total of two whole days in Chicago, but it was worth it to see our families. We were engaged to be married and living together, so each of our families warmly welcomed us. The difference between our families is striking. My family are small talkers, warm, and affectionate. My mom asked Jess all the questions, wanting to know what life was like living with me in California. When we got to Jess's family's house, no questions. They aren't big on small talk, but they can clear out an entire gathering room during family reunions due to their collective gas production. They also have a lovely Christmas tradition of opening presents starting with the youngest grandchild and moving upwards by age to the oldest, Jess's dad.

I'd brought my laptop so I could program for Heidi on the road. I didn't bring my 18x24 season planning canvas, but I did take a picture of it. I referenced it as I sat down at the kitchen table in Jess's parent's house after bumming an internet password from her mother on Sunday before heading home.

After just a few lighter volume days, Heidi miraculously felt better already. I could not believe it. When I began to feel overtraining effects as an athlete, it took me almost two weeks of lower volume work to feel mentally clear and physically ready again. Heidi bounced back as quick as a jackrabbit. For that week, I wrote her some moderately tough PT training sessions with short rest to stimulate some lactate. Frequently training with high lactate can lead to injury, so I only liked to sprinkle this potent stimulus into her training once or twice a month for specific tasks. She handled it well and wanted more. Her sprinting was coming along as her foot continued to heal, and her hiking was improving quickly.

Each week, I had Heidi complete three hikes. One "quarter-pack" hike, this week with 15 pounds, one "half-pack" hike with 25 pounds, and the heavy-pack training at 53 pounds. Her hiking was progressing well each week. Heidi was still working on her mantras while she hiked, especially during the heavy pack training. She also continued to practice the "raisin meditation" while eating. She noted that she completed this task on 5 out of 7 days that week.

Heidi continued to practice her mantras each week. While mantras are helpful to stimulate some arousal to accomplish challenging tasks, some things demand a stronger elixir. This was the first week that I wrote in "Wim Hof" breathing for her to experiment with. I intended for this tool to help summon a stronger physiological call to action.

With Heidi being a quiet person, I imagined that in the past she would psych herself out and meet challenges somewhat flat at rookie training. Flat, or meek, is not a good way to go into a tough physical event! My hypothesis was that she needed to add some strategies to increase her arousal. Heidi told me some stories about how she had performed during the previous two years of rookie training, which backed up my hypothesis. In her first year, she seemed to lack the physical firepower necessary to stay "up" when the going got tough. This caused her to make mistakes while learning the parachute jump commands and she was washed for it. In the second year, the heavy pack test got her on day one. Not fast enough, and out she went. This time around, to help Heidi combat this "flatness," I suggested that she test out "Wim Hof"-style breathing before and during her more challenging training sessions throughout the week. She practiced this with such frequency that it became her go-to for increasing arousal and aligning her mind and body.

Wim Hof breathing is a style of breathwork that upregulates sympathetic nervous system function through hyperventilation. This specific style is similar to ancient Tummo breathing, which dates back to texts from the eighth century.

To perform Wim Hof or Tummo-style breathing, lie on your back in a safe place and begin taking large and fast inhales and exhales. You can set a timer for a minute or two of this. At the end of a cycle of breaths, exhale all the air out of your lungs and hold until the desire to breathe returns.

With practice, it is possible to hold one's breath for 3–4 minutes on an exhale after a few cycles of this breathing pattern.

Heidi would incorporate hard and fast inhales and exhales to help sharpen her mindset and allow her control of her arousal level, on the spot. This type of breathing helped her upregulate arousal by increasing adrenaline. Heidi practiced this specific breathwork multiple times a week as a precursor to

Coaching a quiet athlete can be a starkly contrasting experience compared to someone who is overconfident or brash. Ultimately, it comes down to helping your athlete meet stressors head-on. The quiet athletes seem to have trouble summoning enough arousal to meet big, scary challenges. The loud athlete has no problem here but may falter on a finely detailed task because they bring in too much arousal for the demands of the situation. I look at this through the simple lens of "uppers" and "downers," like the mushrooms from Alice in Wonderland. If someone is too short (the quiet athlete), they need an upper. That's where mantra practice and incorporation of Wim Hof comes in handy. If an athlete is too large (the loud athlete), they need a downer. That's where calming activities like yoga nidra, mindfulness meditation, and visualization are useful.

challenging tasks during training. We were using this frequently to build confidence with the strategy so Heidi would understand and know how and when to use this during rookie training.

After a single session practicing the Wim Hof method, Heidi was hooked. Breath holding was not a strong skill for her. I found this out through her feedback in the sheets! At first, she could only hold her breath on an inhale for 0:37 seconds. After a single Wim Hof session, she noted, "I could easily hold for 1 min without even struggling! That was crazy." I learned a significant piece of information from her feedback—her breathing needed work. I could not believe how poor Heidi's breathing ability was despite her impressive running ability. A recreational athlete can hold their breath for at least a minute. Better athletes can hold their breath for closer to two minutes, and top athletes for over three. Perhaps improving Heidi's breathing was a crucial lever that we hadn't yet experimented with!

Knowing how much Wim Hoff-ing to do (and when) became an important weekly practice for Heidi. This taught her a valuable lesson about spending "arousal dollars." If she spent all her adrenaline on one single task or during one single day of training, then the next task or day she'd feel depleted and unable to summon enough arousal to combat the next day's challenges. Learning to summon just enough arousal to meet the task at hand is crucial. Heidi diligently practiced this breathing strategy each week.

Self-guided titration of arousal is summed up in sport science as Performance Arousal Theory, which is also referred to as the Inverted U model of arousal due to the shape of the curve when the theory is graphed. I like to call the shape an arch instead of an inverted U because an arch has two sides that uphold it, and the center piece on top, the keystone, keeps the arch from crumbling. The theory suggests that performance is optimized at an intermediate level of arousal, at the top of the inverted U, or in my explanation, the top of the arch. Overarousal stimulates too much adrenaline and not enough motor and cognitive control. An athlete operating here would be on the far right end of the graph where arousal is very high and performance is sub-optimal. Underarousal fails to stimulate an appropriate response to

Arousal in sports refers to the level of activation and alertness of the athlete. When an athlete feels excitement AND/OR nervousness before a competition, adrenaline is the molecule that causes this feeling. When arousal levels are low, so is adrenaline. When arousal levels are high, so is adrenaline.

If arousal is too low, an athlete may feel "flat" and seem meek or quiet. To the contrary, if arousal is too high, an athlete may be very activated and alert, perhaps to the point at which they can no longer execute fine motor skills.

Success in some sporting events, like sinking a putt in golf, require low (and yet very specific) level of arousal and adrenaline. Conversely, a sport like powerlifting where an athlete attempts a maximally heavy deadlift requires the highest level of adrenaline in sport. There is relatively low skill in a deadlift, so adrenaline can be very high without negative consequences. The match-winning putt, however, goes past the hole or amiss if adrenaline is a hair too high!

This happened to me once in a decathlon. As a young decathlete, you only get to complete in two or three full decathlons during a single collegiate track season, which puts a ton of pressure on the athlete to perform well at each rare opportunity. Any more frequently than that, and your body breaks down, and you never reach your peak.

The decathlon begins with the 100-meter dash, followed by the long jump. In this particular decathlon, the weather was perfect, and I was PUMPED up that day. Mike had me experiment with a shorter warm-up, and I felt great. I ran the fastest 100-meter of my life and went into the long jump in full arousal. I ended up jumping a full two feet shorter than my best mark. I was too jazzed up. My mark was off because I was running too fast, and my rhythm was off because I was straining too hard. Lesson learned. Arousal is a delicate element, and each athlete must learn to master themselves, matching their arousal to the task at hand.

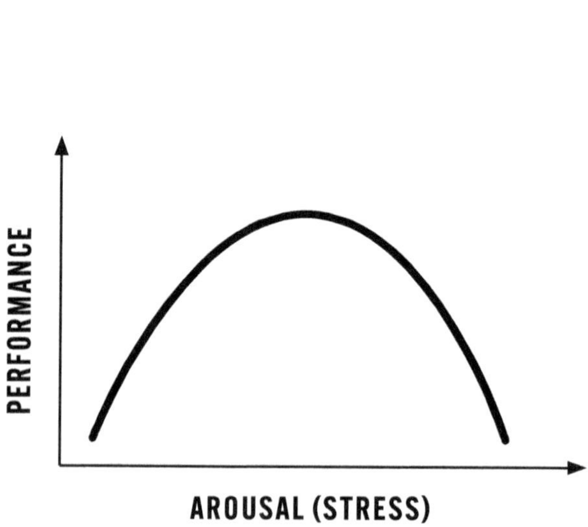

the situation. An athlete's arousal and performance in this state could be graphed on the left side near the y-axis, and their performance would also be suboptimal.

The central nervous system plays a crucial role in arousal. There are two branches of the autonomic nervous system—parasympathetic and sympathetic. The parasympathetic nervous system is for recovery tasks. Eating, sleep, and sex are enabled when this branch of the nervous system is dominant. The sympathetic nervous system is our aggression zone. Actions that demand an increased heart rate and blood flow stimulate the sympathetic nervous system.

Each physiological task that we undergo falls somewhere on the dominance spectrum of sympathetic to parasympathetic. Both systems cannot function maximally at the same time. Either system is the dominant operator at any one point in time, and we can also create a state where we straddle the line between them. Toggling between these two systems in real time, right on the divide, is a state referred to as flow. Flow is the most useful state for athletes (and humans, I argue) because here we precariously sit atop the performance arousal arch, living in the moment. This is where performance in anything that requires high cognitive or fine motor skill is maximized.

At the end of this training week, Heidi competed in the San Diego holiday 5k and won. She wrote, "Fun!! 20:44 was my time. 1st female & 9th overall, small race. Good cause, they got over 400 toys for the toy drive! Total of 5.5 miles today with the warm-up & cool down." Even though I wasn't a fan of Heidi racing during training season, she seemed to enjoy the challenge, it was for a good cause, and it also seemed to re-spark her competitiveness that she had been lacking for the past month. She was back in business.

MONDAY, JANUARY 2, 2017 (16 WEEKS OUT)

Out with 2016, and in with 2017. New Year's Eve came and went. Jess and I rang in the new year at a party with friends from her degree program. We drank, played games, ate a bunch of appetizers, reluctantly took shots of fireball, and slept there at the house. It was a welcomed break from the rigidity of my coaching and master's program. When they asked how I was doing and what I was up to, I told them about Heidi, my newest smokejumper hopeful and what she had ahead of her for training and selection. This fired up some of the group. Later that evening, long after we had rung in the new year with a slurred countdown, messy toasts, drunken promises for the new year, and a few more shots of fireball, a push-up contest broke out, inspired by Heidi's challenge! Jess doesn't like push-ups because they bother her shoulder, so she found a place under some stairs and ripped off a few strict pull-ups instead. When Jess drinks, pull-ups are her go-to.

There were some impressive drunken performances on the impromptu PT test, but no one came close to Heidi's current maxes. It may sound doable to complete 80+ push-ups in a single set without breaking plank or completing more than 15 pull-ups. However, the quality of each repetition must be sound and consistent. When I watch most people do push-ups, the reps get ugly after 20. For Heidi, the quality of her push-ups had to be good enough to count at rookie training. If her chest didn't get low enough on some reps, those push-ups wouldn't count. If her chin didn't make it over the bar, or if she failed to lock her elbows out at the bottom of each rep, the pull-up wouldn't count. Quality matters, and so she trained with that in mind.

Heidi and I started off the new year well. We now communicated smoothly back and forth through the spreadsheet and texts, and sometimes we hopped on a call to iron out more detailed solutions to situations that arose.

Thursday: Heavy Pack Training:
3 miles, ~63–65 lbs., for time

Heidi's feedback: "Afternoon training (waited about 3 hours between). 65 lb. 56 min. Mentally tough today, pack feeling heavier."

My response: "Ok. Good job. Great feedback. I've been waiting for the pack to feel heavy. I'll keep the same pack weight for next week and see how you adapt."

Up until this point, Heidi had been training in her basement in Forest Falls. In place of a staircase was a wooden ladder that led straight down next to her laundry chute. Just like Heidi, her training environment was all function and no nonsense. Her basement was dark and cold. She had a barbell and some plates, a rower, some dumbbells, a jump rope, and a medicine ball. This week, she bought some five and two-point-five-pound plates and a squat rack. I had asked her to purchase those "change plates," as they are called, so that we could get more detailed with weight jumps on her barbell movements. Her home gym was now complete, minus the Rocky posters. Instead, she had an old running trophy and a washer/dryer.

Going forward, we relied on swimming to help Heidi increase training time. Heidi was a strong swimmer (of courses she was). Swimming is great for adding cardiorespiratory load because it's low impact. Most of the time, I asked Heidi to treat her swimming sessions like active recovery, working at a very easy pace. My hope was that she would leave feeling better than she felt beforehand. This is a sure sign of a "tonic" workout, one that rejuvenates the body and mind.

Heidi was now training 14–16 hours a week. Her pack training was coming along well. She now rucked with 65 pounds for three somewhat flat miles, finishing in 50 minutes—plenty of padding there below her 65-minute goal. However, we still had 45 pounds of resistance to add during the next few months.

Heidi also let me know that we needed to fit in her first PT test so that she could submit those scores to the rookie trainers at Boise. They only required scores in max push-ups, pull-ups, sit-ups, and 1.5 mile run time. She said there are only three PT tests between now and her start date. The first PT test was now scheduled only a short week and a half away!

MONDAY JANUARY 9, 2017 (15 WEEKS OUT)

Through each month as the start date of rookie training approached, Heidi steadily improved. She informed me that from here out the rookie trainers at the Boise base had asked her to submit PT scores every few weeks. I reluctantly wrote her first PT test that week. A max set of dead hang pull-ups, a max set of push-ups without breaking plank, three minutes to collect a maximum number of anchored sit-ups, and a 1.5-mile run, for time. During this week, her maxes were solid:

	BLM High Standards	*Heidi's January Maxes*	*Heidi's Initial Goals*
1.5-mile Run	9:30	9:22	9:00
Pull-ups	10	17	20
Push-ups	35	70	85
Sit-ups	60	116	130
Pack Test	110 lbs., 3 miles, 65:00	70 lbs., 3 miles, 55:30	110 lbs., 3 miles, 65:00

I hate testing my athletes until it's absolutely necessary. I work to teach my athletes to embrace the training progressions and to fall in love with the process. This is a rinse and repeat conversation because most athletes misunderstand this concept the first few go-arounds. Sometimes grasping the "it takes time for your body to adapt" approach takes months or years to permeate some of the thick skulls I coach.

Testing is fun because you get to "see" the results of your training and what your body is capable of, but when you test, you show your cards. Testing is not training. And each time you test, you expend energy that could have been used to further prepare you. Testing is depleting, and training, the opposite. In my opinion, most of the time, when not competing (in the case of rookie smokejumpers, "competing" occurs at rookie training), an athlete's time should be spent in preparation for the competition.

When you challenge your body to produce a maximum repetition set to test what you are capable of, you sacrifice a day of progressive training. Progressive training is what enables the ability to hit big numbers come testing day, while creating the capacity to withstand all the other demands of rookie training! Testing is also risky. Athletes don't often get injured from a routine training day. They are much more likely to tweak something when testing or pushing their intensity. I realized the rookie trainers desired this information to ensure that each candidate was progressing and likely to show up physically ready for rookie training, but that didn't mean I had to like it.

A volume-building training day for Heidi at this time worked at 5–10 pull-ups, 15–30 push-ups, and sets of 25–65 sit-ups per set.

Heidi's heavy pack test training load was now up to 70 pounds, and she completed two rounds of 1.5 miles with a 10-to-15-minute rest between bouts. Total work time was 55:30. Not bad! The heavy pack weight was beginning to creep up towards her bodyweight, and this began to feel heavy. Instead of going three straight miles from here, I planned to break the training up into 3 rounds of one mile for the first week at one weight, then in the second week, two rounds of 1.5 miles. The third week at the same weight would be the full three miles, unbroken. The following week, we'd increase pack weight. Heidi loved this approach because the 10-15 minute break between bouts was replenishing enough to keep her speed right where we wanted it to be. She needed to go sub-65 minutes on the first day of rookie training, or else she would wash again.

Training: Heavy Pack Training: 2 Rounds: 1.5 mile walk, ~70 lbs., each for time. Rest 10-15 minutes between rounds.

Details/comments: "This is how I plan to build your volume with heavy packs! Split it up into interval training. Thoughts?"

Heidi: "Sounds great! I can only get stronger!! I love this approach. YEEHAW! Round 1 done 27:00. Round 2, 28:33 I didn't feel slower though... I actually felt strong today and shuffled my lil heart out poncho on in the pouring rain! But felt great! Note: any ankle strengthening stuff? They burn on those steep hikes and the pack test of calves are sore. I guess hiking and yoga huh? They do feel pretty strong ..."

Me: "LOL I can now see you shuffling away in my mind. I'll put some calve-strengthening work in for you. Good times on this!!"

I could tell from her splits how adequate the rest break was. Her splits this week were 27:00 and 28:33, the second 1.5 miles a mere 5% slower than the first. This was perfect and was a good sign that Heidi would be ready the next week for the full three miles with no break. If she fell off on the second interval to 15–20% slower, then that would be a clear sign that we either jumped the pack weight too high that week, or that she was bogged down with recovering from her other training and needed a week deload. So far, so good!

During this carry, Heidi noted that her calves and ankles are getting fatigued. This was the first time that she had mentioned this to me, so I wrote back to her through the sheets that I'd add in some specific lower leg training moving forwards. The following week, I planned to add jump rope and calf raises.

In addition to shoring up weakness in her lower legs, Heidi continued to work on improving her mindset. We utilized every percentage point that we could garner to help optimize her training and recovery. This week, she worked up to 25–30 minutes of the "UCLA body scan meditation," a unique guided meditation that she found one day while digging around online. This was a soundtrack that she utilized to help downregulate her nervous system to improve her recovery. This served dual purposes by also improving her visualization and connection between her mind and body, allowing her to further dig down into parasympathetic stimulation. Heidi practiced these body scan meditations either midday or at night before bed.

Body scan meditations are very similar to yoga nidra, which dates back 1000 years BCE. In 2023, yoga nidra, which is a type of non-steep deep rest (NSDR), is currently being studied extensively for its effects on health, stress reduction, and recovery. In 2016, NSDR and yoga nidra research was almost nonexistent. While training Heidi, I was completely unaware of the research. We just knew it worked, and it helped her recover more fully, and faster. Often anecdotal experiences prove powerful when studied, but the research can take many years to expand into widespread use.

MONDAY JANUARY 16, 2017 (14 WEEKS OUT)

Heidi is an extremely competitive athlete. To leverage this to our advantage for maximizing training opportunities, Heidi said she wanted to sign up for some competitions throughout her training season to test herself. The comps also served the purpose of pushing her beyond her comfortable training intensities that she experienced each week while training solo.

The beginning of one week started out well. Heidi was in good spirits. On Monday after her 100-minute hike through the mountains with a light pack weighing 35 lbs., her feedback made me laugh when she wrote, "Amazing hike. Beautiful day. Nothing better than a hike on a sunny day at Del Rosa to perk up a stale spirit. My legs felt like a POWER HOUSE! A little sore from strength today but that subsided as I pushed hard! Hikes supts hill, bonus, bonus, the one, bonus, bonus, bonus then back side of meatball." I have no idea what any of those hikes are.

Wednesday, Heidi's pack weight was 70 pounds for three straight miles with no break, completed in 56:30. This is a fantastic time. She came in only one minute slower than the week before on the 2 x 1.5-mile heavy carry with that 10-minute rest between bouts.

Unfortunately, later during this same week, Heidi began to experience mild overreaching symptoms in the form of psychological distress. I noticed some negativity in her feedback after a simple barbell and medicine ball drill that was very much unlike her usual quirky and chipper responses.

Heidi's feedback: "13:56, very frustrated and angry at myself not keeping the OT2M. My last 2 rounds were the best, even went unbroken on wb. Really down on myself right now, I should be able to do this and I can I just don't know what happened. Am I where I should be? Didn't push myself to keep under 2min so I just would rest and work and rest and not good."

My response: "Interesting! next week we'll deload. What took up the most time—the power cleans or the wallball shots? You are exactly where you should be. Stay positive! For realz. We're fine!!! If I make a mistake and ask too much of you, don't beat yourself up. We've done so much training that a slight deload will make you feel much better! This week is the toughest yet. Hang in there, Heidi."

No happy emojis here. I could feel her frustration, and it made my stomach hurt. These moments as a coach always make you question your methods. It's not uncommon during heavy training blocks for athletes to feel ok at the beginning of the week, and later in that same week, they begin to lose their edge. I learned this as a college athlete and again through the lens of a coach. I knew what it felt like to hit a midweek brick wall. The task is supposed to feel easy, and it doesn't. Or maybe it's downright soul sucking. This can demoralize you and drive you into a downward emotional spiral. Sometimes, an "all is lost" thought pattern sneaks into your head, and it's really challenging to overcome.

Shadowing under Tonja at U of I, I learned that if an athlete isn't performing how you expected, it's ok to pivot midweek, even mid-drill. Since Heidi was following the spreadsheet and completing the training at home without me present, I couldn't simply change the training parameters on the spot to alleviate the situation. Instead, I was a day behind. Now I had to play catch-up.

I tried to calm Heidi down and reframe the situation by stating that she was right where she needed to be. This often helps calm an overactive imagination, one that is fragile from fatigue. I also noted that the next week would be a deload since this was the third week in a row pushing hard. Her training duration for this week was scheduled for 16 hours of work, so next week I planned to drop the volume to stimulate recovery. I had watched Mike follow this protocol at U of I with our jumpers and multi-event athletes just about every month for three years straight. I knew that after the deload week, she would feel physically better, and this would help alleviate much of her mental anguish.

Saturday of this week was her first competition of the training season. I didn't expect much out of Heidi for this race because she had what seemed on paper like a tough week. I wrote this in her sheets, which probably fired her up to run fast. Tell Heidi that she can't do something and see how that goes.

Seemingly to spite me and show that she could run well no matter how tough the week, Heidi finished the Manhattan Beach 5k in 20:24. This was a PR for her. This is about 6:33 mile pace, which showed that her running speed was increasing, and her goal time of holding a 6:00 mile pace was within reach. My logic: if she could hold 3.1 miles (5k) at 6:33 per mile, then she should be able to run faster for the 1.5-mile run where the distanced is less than half!

Later in the same day of her 5k race, she hiked for another two hours at elevation to complete her light pack training with 20 pounds. What a week!

Continuing with my Sunday programming, I spent an increasing amount of time sitting at my big wooden table in my cramped apartment scribbling away on my oversized piece of textured white watercolor paper left over from one of my painting classes at Redlands. I transcribed my plan for Heidi into her spreadsheet. I'm a detail-oriented person and sometimes I have trouble taking a step back to view the big picture, so seeing Heidi's complete year plan laid out on one large piece of paper was extremely helpful. The grand vision has always been elusive to me, so I spent time making sure that her journey from month one to month six was full of everything she needed and nothing she didn't. This kept me from spending too much time playing around with the details, and the painter's paper helped me limit the potential for making a glaring season planning mistake.

I could not afford to miss something important, whether it be an opportunity or a threat to Heidi's immediate or future performance. Each touchpoint with Heidi served as a sieve to expose errors and uncover opportunities. Each time I found an error in her training, I'd get a pang of emotion in my gut, spend time fixing the error, and breathe a sigh of relief, hoping that the correction was optimal. Time would tell the following week when Heidi completed the training on her own and typed in her feedback for me to review.

MONDAY, JANUARY 23, 2017 (13 WEEKS OUT)

After Heidi's small mindset break, I deloaded her total training volume. Over the previous three weeks, her weekly training hours went from 14 hours to 15, then we peaked at 16 hours the week before, and we dropped back down to 13 hours this week. Deload weeks are my favorite time to add in new tasks. This allows the athletes to acclimate to the new demands with a lower number of reps, distance, or duration. The changes this week looked challenging.

Now that we were approaching three months out from rookie training, it felt like the right time to become more specific with training some of the actual scenarios that Heidi might experience in Boise. Up until this point, we had been working to improve tasks individually. Hiking, running, PT, and strength and power training sessions had all been separate. Now, it was time to begin combining these together into larger chunks of work.

For Monday's "half-pack" training (I call this day half-pack because the weight is about half of her heavy pack training day, this week 45 pounds), Heidi completed a short 2.5-mile hike in Forest Falls, in snowshoes. The difference this week was at three different points in the hike, she stopped and completed hello dollies, flutters, and glute bridges. This took her just over an hour.

Even though it was a lower volume training week, it was time to bump up Heidi's heavy pack weight. To introduce the increase from 70 to 80 pounds, I split up the training into three sets of one mile, each with 10 minutes of rest. This was a big weight jump for her, and she finished each mile in 21 minutes for a total work duration of 63 minutes, which pushed up dangerously close to that 65-minute mark. This worried both of us. Her feedback expressed a frustrated emoji. However, it wasn't all bad. Part of the result came from her route. She was training at elevation, and there was snow on the ground. This was true for most of her training so far. Heidi was running and hiking in the snow near her home, over one mile above sea level. I would joke with Jess that

Heidi was a female version of "Rocky," rucking and running around the snowy mountains with "Eye of the Tiger" blaring, all in preparation for her big fight in Boise against the best men in the fire world. She really was training like a madwoman. There was only one thing that I foresaw slowing her progress. Her feet. After the previous week's 5k race, she later began to experience shin pain while running. I knew this was linked to her foot pain from earlier in the training season, and that numbness was morphing into shin pain. This was not good.

MONDAY, JANUARY 30, 2017 (12 WEEKS OUT)

Heidi mentioned a massive knot in her quads. Her shins were still tender as well. The week before, I was hoping that Heidi's shin pain was just a one-off, fleeting pain after her race. Now that she mentioned it two weeks in a row, the alarm bells were going off. "Do you want me to drop your running mileage to allow for shin splints to heal? They are pesky and will get worse as your weekly accumulated running volume increases. My gut tells me to drop your running down to allow for healing, but I like to play the safe route ..." She replied, "I'm good! Doing voodoo (voodoo is a mobility method) & rolling and bath soaks. They are much better! No need to drop mileage yet." Heidi was convinced that her recovery methods would help hold her together and she shouldn't slow down. I planned to keep a close eye out. If she displayed worsening symptoms, I would have to decrease training volume, which Heidi didn't want.

She continued to utilize her mantras and Wim Hof breathing. However, there seemed to be a missing piece to her mindset training. This week, I introduced the most psychologically challenging mental training strategy that we utilized during her preparation—visualization.

Heidi was in a unique position having had rookie training experience from the previous two years. However, this year she was headed to Boise. She had four weeks of rookie training experience from two years ago at McCall and just a single day from Boise last year. Therefore, painting a clear mental picture of how the 5–6 weeks of rookie training at Boise might unfold would be impossible. There were too many unknowns. However, I still believed visualization would be a powerful mindset preparation tool for Heidi. She had anxiety about going back to Boise, and these simple mindset tools could be powerful for bolstering Heidi's self-confidence.

I asked Heidi to conjure up past scenarios or best guess predictions with as much detail as possible—the color of the mountainside in the distance as they hiked, the smell of the dirt as they held push-up planks on a mid-hike PT, the texture of the pine bark and sage as they climbed, the taste of sweat and dust as they cut line, the burning in her legs as she climbed the jump tower with 80 pounds of gear. I asked her to put herself mentally back there, to the most difficult times, and imagine herself overcoming those situations.

Her first imagery feedback on Monday January 30th:

"Felt good. Imagined first morning roll call, pt test and my smooth transitions remaining calm while being yelled at. Breathing. Staying hydrated. Visualized eating a power snack after the calisthenics. Visualized 25pull ups, pushing to exhaustion on push ups, cutting through the air like a knife through butter on sit ups getting 130. Maintaining my calm cool collection, keeping track of time on my watch. Supporting others. The run. Remained calm, wim hoff & warm up. Smooth run under 9:30, then pushing past the pain on that 2nd 1.5 mile. Seeing those ahead of me but knowing I'm in the mix, I'm hitting my time, I'm staying smart. I could feel my heart rate go up but kept breathing and stayed calm. I like this exercise. Successful round #1 for pt test day 1."

This was a great start. When I wrote this drill in for her, I expected her to write, "done," or "check." I did not expect her to describe what she visualized, but I'm glad she did. It gave me an even deeper glimpse into her psyche.

MONDAY, FEBRUARY 6, 2017 (10 WEEKS OUT)

Heidi's mental training was improving quickly. She was getting more detailed with her visualization skills. Each week, I wrote up her mental training assignment at the top of her weekly training sheets:

"Imagery Practice: 10 minutes - Pick a difficult task you might encounter in rookie training and imagine the situation in as much detail as you can. Put yourself there. Once the scene is set, imagine yourself performing the task successfully. Once you can imagine it 5 times in a row successfully, pick another task!"

And here was her response on Monday of that week:

"I went to bed last night thinking about jumping and it was in my dreams and all successful. I am not 100% sure on Blm jump method but I have an idea and that is what I'm rehearsing, just don't want to formulate bad habits or wrong jump count cadence. 5th imagery for pt test. I could feel my nerves, the way my body reacts to nervousness, I could feel the adrenaline coursing through my veins giving me that light headed and bodily tingly feeling. I was first in line for each exercise. Pull ups 21 then started timer for 5min rest with no prompts, 91 push ups, 5 min rest, 145 sit ups. Shook my arms out stretched. Loaded up vans organized kept foot lockers in seats. Driven to park. 10min warm up got my heart rate up with runners warm up. First 1.5 9:13, turn around knock out 1.5 total time 20:45. Remained calm, focused and smooth for all transitions, pack packing, vehicle loading, etc."

I had experienced meditations like this during college track and field. Mike guided our entire team through visualizations like this and took us through a mental journey of our upcoming conference championship as we lay on the ground in a Redlands classroom. Many of my anxious teammates giggled, writhed, and made jokes during this time instead of focusing on conjuring up finely detailed imagery. They did not perform well in the competition. The athletes who took it seriously all set personal best marks. This stuff was powerful. I was excited that Heidi had quickly bought in.

Four weeks had already passed since her first PT test in January. This week was her second opportunity to test. While I still didn't like the idea of testing this frequently, I did enjoy the rush of the experience. Heidi always brought her best effort. She had a tenacity about her. She was going to improve or die trying.

On Thursday February 9, 2017, Heidi met me at the gym and completed a PT test:

	BLM High Standards	*Heidi's January Maxes*	*Heidi's February Maxes (this week)*	*Heidi's Initial Goals*
1.5-mile Run	9:30	9:22	9:16	9:00
Pull-ups	10	17	18	20
Push-ups	35	70	78	85
Sit-ups	60	116	123	130
Pack Test (3.0 miles)	110 lbs., 65:00	70 lbs., 55:30	80 lbs., 54:00!	110 lbs., 65:00

I filmed all her sets so I could watch later and look for technical improvements or places where the rookie trainers might not count some of her repetitions. Overall, she performed great reps. All her marks on this day were personal bests! She was pumped up! I felt high on life after training with her. The plan was working. We were on our way.

Afterwards, I rewatched the videos. I noticed that her sit-up technique still needed work, so I planned to write in sit-up technique sets into her training, along with her maximum speed sit-up work.

At the end of that week, Heidi was tired. On Saturday, she wrote, "3.74 miles soldier hike at Del Rosa. I was tired and mentally did not want to do it, so you know what I did? I said, I'm doing soldier today (steepest, longest one way up hike at Del Rosa) and I had a goal to get to the top & I did :)" I beamed with pride while taking this comment in. This was the type of mindset that she had cultivated through her training and would continue to improve upon as we marched towards rookie training. She was beginning to do what needed to be done no matter how she felt. This placed an even larger burden on my shoulders to program the right amount of training for her. If I programmed too much, she was now becoming mentally strong enough to push through it. This is extremely dangerous. It's also the exact mindset that Heidi would need to push through rookie training—to dig deep and handle whatever was thrown at her, no matter how challenging.

Imagine that an athlete is paying you to help them prepare for something massive, and they have one shot at it. They are passionate, almost desperate, to succeed, and they are relying on you to guide them. If you train them too hard, they go into rookie training at their peak but unrested and full of nagging injuries—small things, mostly. However, this strategy will cause an athlete to completely break when placed under enough pressure. At rookie training, those small injuries turn into full-blown gaskets, and they wash because a broken athlete doesn't last a week in rookie training. Conversely, if you don't push hard enough, they go in underprepared and fail after a few weeks because they don't have capacity to handle the sheer physical volume of work. Once the body goes, the mind follows.

There was a lot on the line for Heidi, and for me. I felt the pressure. When texting Heidi on Sunday that her next week of training was ready, there was an odd sensation gnawing in my stomach. Was I babying her? Was I displacing my own limitations on how much I pushed her? I was afraid to injure her. I had never pushed an athlete this hard before. Even those physical specimens at Illinois, some of them who went on to the Olympics in track and field and bobsled, they never trained with this much work. Heidi's training volume was insanely high, and yet I felt that it might not be enough. Rookie training would be more than 5 weeks of physical work, each week comprised of 40–50 hours of hard work. I believed that if we couldn't reach at least half of that weekly volume in training, then she had a poor chance. So that's what we aimed for: One to two weeks containing 20 hours of work during her peak month, March, which was approaching quickly. Heidi had finished the past week at just shy of 18 training hours. We were close.

MONDAY, FEBRUARY 13, 2017 (9 WEEKS OUT)

Two years before at McCall, Heidi's biggest limitation was the jump tower. Four flights of stairs with over 80 pounds of jump gear at 120 pounds of bodyweight, practicing complex jump cadences for hours on end. This week we began specific preparation for the jump tower by loading Heidi up with a pack or a barbell and having her perform higher volume low box step-ups. I had so much planned, a week packed with heavy and long hikes and grueling training, a ton of PT, and 19 hours of training. It was the week of Valentine's Day. In Heidi's sheets I aptly titled it The Valentine's Week Massacre, because it looked brutal on paper. Consider that some training sessions look easy on paper and are rough when tackled. Therefore, things that look tough on paper are usually much, much worse.

On Wednesday during this week, Heidi fell off some of the intra-workout targets that I had set for her. I sat in the kitchen slumped over with my elbows on the table, face pressed between my palms, and staring into my computer pondering what to do. No upbeat, funny comments. No emojis. She was beginning to spin out. As soon as I read her feedback, I knew that we had to pull back. She had skipped swimming and yoga one day because she was tired, and she was not happy about the skipped ("failed") workouts. This was very unlike her. Later this same day, she showed up to the track for her interval training and got kicked off. A perfect negative shitstorm brewed. After this, at the gym,

I programmed the barbell lunges too heavy, and she just lost it. "Wow my legs are not confident on this :/ I could barely do 70 lbs. :(not good. I think if I can get better at these, I'll be better hiking the heavy weight? Weak & wobbly. I feel like rookie training is fast approaching ..." This was worry-speak in Heidi language. I felt like she needed a week off, but we didn't have the time.

To top it all off, the shin splints seemed to be getting worse. How could we build her running volume with her shin splints flaring up?! We couldn't. What if she arrived at rookie training with her shins a mess? She wouldn't make it. Ugh. I thought to myself, *why did I push her hard two weeks in a row?* Noticing my despair, Jess took a quick break from her studies and decided to cheer me up. "Uhh-hu-hu-hu." I looked up to see Jess standing in the middle of the living room with her sweatpants pulled up almost to her chest, with her back rounded, belly puffed out and slightly nodding her head. By the odd look on her face, I thought she might be having a stroke. I lifted my eyebrows and said, "What are you d-" She interrupted even louder, "UHHHH-hu-hu!"

I smiled, catching the game. She was performing her Lorraine impression from Mad TV! I began to play back, throwing out simple questions which she immediately batted down with "Yeah-ya-ya-ya-UHHH-hu-hu." By the end, we were laughing hysterically, and the stress of the moment was gone.

Afterwards, in better spirits, I decided to decrease her training volume and lighten the weight on the rest of her tasks for the rest of the week. I hoped that it would be enough recovery to prepare her for what was about to come.

MONDAY, FEBRUARY 20, 2017 (8 WEEKS OUT)

We had eight weeks before Heidi began rookie training at Boise. I experienced many firsts while working with Heidi, and perhaps the most important and terrifying experience in her preparation was planning this final two months of her training. Up until this point, I would plan only a few weeks ahead, and the planning would be loose. I did this purposefully to leave some wiggle room to adjust training volume and other programming variables depending on how Heidi responded to the increases in volume. I kept the overall season progression in mind and attempted to stay on it, but the details each week changed frequently depending on her feedback.

From here forwards, I wanted to be more specific with planning Heidi's training targets as we moved towards her peak week (the highest training volume in a single week), which looked like it was going to be the last week of March, Week 22. By now, I had a good idea of what Heidi was capable of. I also had a decent feel for her recovery ability and potential, so I gave myself ample time to sit down at the kitchen table with her season plan and sketch out the ideal finishing periodization structure for the upcoming eight weeks.

I drew inspiration and direction from a few sources. First, my personal experience as a college athlete. Second, from my experience at U of I as I watched Tonja and Mike prepare their athletes for the national championships each year. And third, I used my research ability honed through my two master's degrees and dug into scholarly research on peaking and tapering to help me get laser specific about how to manipulate volume and intensity over the final eight weeks. With these three sources of information on tapering and peaking, I was excited to test my plan out on Heidi. I was also terrified! Heidi was my first athlete with no outside influence, so if she did well, that would be on us. If she failed, that would also be on us. I really hoped that my personal experiences and research would pay off.

I uncovered a handful of peer reviewed scientific studies and articles about tapering. After searching article titles and skimming abstracts, I found one that seemed to contain the information that I was looking for! Olympic female gymnasts. In the study, they compared the effect of a taper on overreached and normally trained athletes, and their data clearly showed that after a period of overload (overreaching), the taper was more effective and produced a much higher level of performance. The data was very specific as well, highlighting a 45% decrease in training volume over 22–30 days. So that's what I planned.

I introduced a new mindset principle to Heidi—flow. I suggested that Heidi begin a narrowing of her of focus on each individual task to help bring her fully into the moment with no worries about the future and no frustration from the past. I told her about where I learned this. A few years before, I listened to a wonderful opening keynote speech at the 2014 NSCA National Conference in Las Vegas. The speaker was a former Navy Seal lieutenant named Pete Scobell. One of his main takeaways during BUD/S (Basic Underwater Demolition/SEAL Training) was that many of the successful seals, including himself, focused on making it through the current set of log sit-ups. Making it to the next break. Making it to lunch. To dinner. To bed. And when things got really tough, simply focusing on making it to the next rep on a seemingly never-ending set of push-ups. Completely living in the moment. Heidi immediately gravitated to like this concept and exclaimed, "Yesss! That's what they say at rookie training too haha!"

The concept of "flow" is the feeling of losing oneself in the moment. Flow is a desirable state for creatives like musicians, artists, and athletes. One cannot summon flow. You can set the stage for it, but flow must find you. As soon as you notice that you're in flow, you are no longer in flow because you are now noticing and not experiencing. A good personal example of this: I love to hike up a mountain trail and then run back down it. I wear those weird toe shoes, and they don't have much of a sole, so when wearing them, I feel every bit of texture on the trail. If I step on a rock, it hurts. So, when I run down the mountain, I must watch exactly where I place each footstep, to the centimeter. If I think "step there, there, and there," I will slip or fall or step on a sharp rock. I won't move as quickly compared to when I turn off my thinking brain and surrender into the moment. Here is where the brain, mind, and body become one. The moment on the mountain becomes all there is. This is the essence of flow.

During the next two months, I had some wild training planned for Heidi. She would need every bit of grit that she could muster. For the week, I had scheduled 16 hours of training, a metric ton of PT tasks, three different hikes, including her heavy pack training (which was now at 90 pounds), close to 30 miles of running, strength training, and rehab exercises. It looked intense, and things were only going to get tougher from here over the next month. The peak month was here!

Heid's visualization continued to improve. She wrote, "110lb pack test. A little chilly in the morning, feel the cold humid air, at the starting line, 3-2-1 go. Shuffling shuffling. Some pull away but I always keep everyone in sight. I am focused on my breathing & on my shuffling. I'm wearing my gps watch and maintaining good time. I have a system, shuffle for a 1/4 mile then long walking strides for 30sec. I can feel the weight, but my body can do this. My legs, core, and mental capacity are stronger. I stay positive, I can do this! I make the half way point at 30min. I continue to shuffle and breathe. My breathing is heavy but steady and methodical with the pack test. Last 1/4 mile I can push it in! My rookie bro's & sis's are with me. I did it. And I can continue the full day of whatever they throw at us."

Heidi crushed her heavy pack test that week. She wrote, "Yeehaw!!!!!! Mile 1 17:19 then realized I was missing 5 lbs., no buggy. So last 2 miles have 90 lbs. But I felt great!! Mentally and physically!!! I believe in myself!! Mile 2 17:30 boom confidence!! Mitochondria!!!! Mile 3 17:36 woo 52:25 total??? Stretchy time! I did pack test before everything else today, lead rookie trainer Staab said I should be able to do it first thing one morning ..." That was great to hear. If Heidi tested this first thing in the morning while fresh, she should be fine. And her mindset during these carries was a breath of fresh air! She was already having success with flow.

MONDAY, FEBRUARY 27, 2017 (7 WEEKS OUT)

Heidi had been in constant contact with the rookie trainers. She had found out that she would be one of two females out of 13 total rookies this year. The experience was becoming more real each week, and so was her visualization. She wrote, "The Plane. First man in stick jump imagery practice. I am nervous! I feel butterflies (for real), my heart is beating out my chest, my throat has a clog. The plane is loud, the spotter and one trainer are shouting above the noise. We are all suited up in our yellow bulky jump suits, our chutes are on our backs and reserves are resting on our knees, we are shoulder to shoulder and hip to hip smooshed on the bench seat facing out the windows. All I see is sky, blue sky and white whispy clouds. We put our helmets on and snap our face masks. I take deep yoga breaths, the blood is pumping so hard in my veins. The first 2-man stick is up. I hear the spotter pointing out the jump spot and trainers on the ground and the yards of drift, only 50yards of drift so light winds. The spotter yells to get in the door, 1st jumper in the door, 'get ready!' Slap, he's out the door, 30" later 2nd jumper is out the door and I have a sudden wave of calmness (for real it was weird). A couple more 2-man sticks go, then im up. Blood pumping again, deep breaths, a little light headed. Spotter ensures I understand the yards of drift and jump spot. 'On final get in the door' I get into the door smooth, efficient, controlled. I am siting on my padded butt , feet outside plane on step. 'Get ready!' Boom I'm poised and ready like a coiled spring hands slapped against outside of plane, core is fired up, slight curve in back ... slap! Boom all my might I have very strong and forceful vigor out the door, pushing off with hands and feet at the same time, powerful exit. Then I'm in the air doing my jump cadence free falling (when I learn the exact cadence at camp for this base I'll continue doing imagery) a slight jolt backward as the canopy opens, look up and check for any malfunctions in the red, blue & white rectangular shoot. I see the sky, feel the cool air. I locate my jump partner and the spot & with smooth toggle movements navigate efficiently to the spot with a smooth soft landing."

I responded, "This is awesome. I can picture this well! I'm sure you are almost physically there, because mentally you're definitely there!! You are getting deep into the imagery. It's difficult to conjure emotions with imagery of a future task and even more difficult to control them. If you can control them now, you're planting seeds that will allow control of them later!"

Notice the level of detail here. At McCall, these scenarios proved problematic due to the difficulty of learning complex motor and cognitive tasks through physical and mental exhaustion. Heidi was relentless and practiced to win. Whenever I saw this type of feedback in her sheets, I knew that she was feeling good. She was dialed in.

I compared Heidi's current stage in training to the athletes I knew best, track and field sprinters, hurdlers, and multi-event athletes. From observing three years of Tonja and Mike preparing some of the best athletes in the country (and a few of the best runners in the world), I thought Heidi was right where she needed to be at this point in the season.

Here is a single training day from this week (19 out of 25), just two weeks away from her peak week:

- 10 minutes of Imagery practice (above): imagine a difficult situation at rookie training with as much detail as possible (colors, wind, foliage, smells, textures, emotions, other people, pain, fatigue, etc.) and execute your tasks well. Once 5 repetitions of the specific task are successfully executed, move on to a different task.
- Explosive 15-minute dynamic warm-up
- 15 minutes of sprint 30m, walk back recovery (23 reps)
- 60 strict pull-ups with boots on, 210 push-ups, 330 sit-ups, and a mile and a half of 400-meter intervals.
- 440 repetitions of core and glute muscle endurance tasks
- 7 mile easy-paced run

- Usually Monday called for a 90 to 120-minute pack hike. This week should have been 60 lbs. for 90 minutes, but it rained and the trails were dangerously muddy. Instead to keep work capacity within the required realm, I had her perform a 45-minute AMRAP of 1000m row + 20 bodyweight squats + 15 burpees. She completed 6+ rounds.
- 3 Rounds of stability work consisting of:
  - High rep hip banded and loaded lunges
  - Glute marching
  - Bench pinch planks—highly recommended to provide Adduction strength and internal hip stability, and are also initially brutally difficult to execute correctly
  - Weighted calf raises to help with ascending steep mountainous terrain.
  - Complete stretch and foot care follows each bout of training each day, sometimes multiple times (30–60 minutes)

This was Heidi's training day 1 of 6 for the 19th week. Each day of her week was difficult, and no days or tasks were repeated. Every running workout was different in intention, speed, and terrain. This specific day was 4 hours of physical work. Over the past four months, she earned the right to train for many hours a day, and she woke up the next morning feeling good enough to conquer another 3–4 more hours of quality work.

I also had Heidi running fast twice a week, one day of sprinting and another day of interval training. The purpose of both days was to help push her running speed faster so she could broach the 9:00 mark on the 1.5-mile run during the PT test. When you are 5 foot 2, you can't just show up and run fast after pounding the pavement running long slow distance. You must also work fast running into the program. The problem with adding in sprints and fast intervals to a training program that's already brimming with training volume is that the risk of injury rachets up a few notches. Heidi's shins were still questionable.

The traditional model of periodization comes from 1950–1980s Russian sport scientists. They hypothesized and tested numerous periodization strategies, eventually arriving at the model many coaches rely on today to peak their athletes. Imagine a line on a graph representing training volume. The line climbs upwards, steadily increasing throughout a training season, peaking near the middle to end of the season, and then decreasing smoothly into the season finale, the culmination event, the Olympics or World Championships. Now add another line onto your graph, this one representing intensity. Throughout the season, intensity climbs but does not increase beyond volume until that middle/end of the graph. Just as volume begins to drop down towards the season finale, that's the crucial point when the intensity line crosses the volume line, increasing through the end of the training cycle. As volume decreases, intensity peaks. The most risk in the entire training cycle is the point where those two lines intersect. Heidi and I were about to pass through that crucial junction.

With the increased risk during this period in training, I suggested that Heidi double down on her recovery modalities. What goes up must also come down. This saying holds true not just for projectiles, but also for emotions and arousal. Athletes can upregulate their bodies to match the physiological demands. Athletes must also demonstrate a heightened ability to relax, or they risk burning out.

To illustrate the concept of the speed of relaxation, picture a novice boxer and a Golden Glove champion. When novices throw punches, they might be completely tense for each punch they throw. However, the Golden Glove champion can be loose in the ring, even while throwing punches. The best boxers and martial artists remain relaxed and quick with strikes until milliseconds before the moment of impact. That's when muscular tension peaks to connect the athlete's fist with the root source of the punch's power, the ground, channeled through the body. Complete tension from fist to ground for a single perfectly harmonized instant allows for a maximally powerful and efficient punch, one that can be thrown multiple times without subsequent decrease in power. The moment after impact, back to complete relaxation. The novice expends much more energy on each strike, fatiguing quickly, power dropping noticeably after each exertion.

How does this apply to training? Tension, then relaxation, that's how! Relaxation is a skill, and skills are trainable. I could teach Heidi to relax more effectively! Keeping one's body aroused all day is impractical and leads to burnout.

In the 5–6 weeks of rookie training, success does not hinge solely on arriving in peak condition. How athletes recover as they trek through the selection process is more important. I suggested that Heidi double-down on her UCLA body scan meditation to help her downregulate. She was approaching her culmination event—the start of rookie training. Imagine her difficulty falling asleep each night as day one crept closer. Furthermore, imagine making it through that first day of rookie training and trying to fall asleep that night after a nerve-filled and adrenaline-packed day! Practicing and building confidence with relaxation strategies would prove immeasurably useful to her. She needed to learn to stay loose between hard punches.

For the first time rookies, ignorance is bliss. Each day of rookie training is a surprise. They only heard stories of what lay ahead. For Heidi, she had some idea, and this tested her mettle. How many times have you done something challenging that you would never do again if you had known better? Heidi was walking back into the flames for a third and final time.

For the rest of her preparation, Heidi frequently practiced downregulation breathing in addition to her mantras and Wim Hof-ing to maximize relaxation and recovery. After intense training sessions, I would have Heidi follow some specific breathing protocols with breath holds and long exhales, combined with calming, relaxing music, the kind that you'd hear while getting a massage. Together these elements work well to decrease arousal, stimulate the parasympathetic system, and initiate recovery. This also provided an opportunity to teach her body and mind to trust these drills.

MONDAY, MARCH 6, 2017 (6 WEEKS OUT)

Smack dab in the middle of the peak week, Heidi faced 16 hours of training, complete with a 90-pound pack carry, which she completed in 58:48. We still trained strength for just shy of 90 minutes this week. We piled on the miles through running, rowing, biking, and swimming. It was a hiking deload this week with only two and a half hours programmed with one light 90-minute hike and the heavy pack training.

The next week she was set to hike for over three and a half hours. To balance her stress equation and act as a buffer to mitigate some of the negative side effects of overreaching, Heidi completed almost four hours of yoga this week along with continued pursuit of mindset changes through practicing her raisin meditation, body scans, breathwork, mantras, and Wim Hof during tough training tasks. Heidi's visualization continued to improve.

And just like that, another month had flown by. It was already time for Heidi's third PT test. She met me at the gym at 10 a.m. after I finished coaching my morning classes, and she got warmed up and ready. We only met like this in person a handful of times, once a month for her monthly PT test. The rest of our interactions were through spreadsheets and cell phone. This morning, Heidi got after it.

	BLM High Standards	*Heidi's January Maxes*	*Heidi's February Maxes*	*Heidi's March Maxes*	*Heidi's Initial Goals*
1.5-mile Run	9:30	9:22	9:16	9.06	9:00
Pull-ups	10	17	18	20	20
Push-ups	35	70	78	95	85
Sit-ups	60	116	123	132	130
Pack Test (3 miles)	110 lbs., 65:00	70 lbs., 55:30	80 lbs., 54:00!	90 lbs., 58:48	110 lbs., 65:00

The remarkable part about her testing today was that she surpassed the goals that she had set for herself at the beginning of the season. The only goals that she didn't yet best were the run and heavy pack test. It was time to set new goals! She set her next pull-up, push-up, and sit-up goals at 22, 100, and 140 reps. We had reached her original goals a month early!

MONDAY, MARCH 13, 2017 (5 WEEKS OUT)

Now that Heidi was ready to crush the PT Test, we could turn our focus towards preparing for hiking with exercises. One of the challenges that rookie trainers put rookies through at McCall was rucking for hours through the forest on steep trails, at elevation, and stopping every so often to "rest" with mid-hike brutal exercise sequences. During a single hike, they might stop multiple times to complete bodyweight exercises or climb trees. To prepare Heidi for this, I began to create mixed hiking and exercise sequences. I instructed her to bring a blanket along on hikes so she could perform ground-based training without getting wet and muddy. I didn't want her to catch a cold. This was the second to last hard training week, and we were pushing right up to the edge. Yep, that theoretical edge I mentioned many pages back. I had written her just shy of 20 training hours this week.

To drive her pull-ups to the next level, this week we began lactate training. I had Heidi utilize hanging-pauses and short rest intervals to accumulate a relatively high volume of work within a short time, which produced a lot of lactate. Although these sessions can be dangerous, Heidi wanted to push her max up another 2 reps, and to do so, she had to dig in further.

Remember when I described the volume and intensity graph? Producing lactate falls far to the right on the graph, beyond that crucial axis point where volume and intensity swap positions. Lactate is produced in high quantities in working muscle tissue when exerting at a rate that greatly exceeds its utilization. While initial lactate research from about 100 years ago dubbed the substrate a waste product and mislabeled it as a factor which slows the rate of physical work, new research from the 1980s and further studies from the early 2000s suggest that lactate is a beneficial substrate that actually helps prolong physical exertion, and as a bonus, is preferentially utilized in brain, heart, and muscle cells. Producing large quantities can be quite uncomfortable, but the training results are often stellar. Just use the stimulus sparingly.

This week, Heidi completed two long hikes with exercises, one on Monday and the second on Friday. The Friday hike:

- Hike with 70lb. Ruck (bring a blanket to do ground-based training & your axe!)
- Hike 40 minutes, then:
  - 3 sets, 15 reps of each: Air Squats, HD's, Glute Bridges, Flutters, Cut Line (15 R/L)
  - Rest 5 minutes
- Hike 30 minutes, then:
  - 3 sets, 15 reps of each: Lunges, Bicycles, Air Squats, HD's, Cut Line (15 R/L)
  - Rest 5 minutes, snack, drink.
- Hike 20 minutes, then:
  - 3 sets, 15 reps of each: Air Squats, HD's, Glute Bridges, Flutters, Cut Line (15 R/L)
- Done.

In between Monday and Friday hikes, for the Wednesday weighted pack training, she completed three rounds of one mile with 100 pounds. We were now just 10 pounds away from her test weight!

On Saturday, she went for a 10-mile easy-paced run, “1 hr 55 min. fun run. PCT east of Baldwin lake in big bear. Sooooo beautiful!! Got some sun too :)” and ended her week with some hip and shoulder mobility and stability work. She took Sunday to rest.

My favorite feedback from this week was a summary of a visualization. Heidi wrote, “I'm not sure I mentioned this before, but what also makes RT (rookie training) hard is short time frames for memorizing and performing suit ups/chute ups, buddy checks, parachute landing falls, let down procedures, jump count, emergency procedures (what to look for and mitigation), let down procedures, etc. We get this information during RT and must memorize verbatim. So, just another mental challenge that I'll practice when I'm there and they give us new information. Imagery practice: hike #3, I feel confident! I see everyone in yellows & greens, QBs over shoulders, bright yellows and greens, hard hats. The mountain slope has flowers blooming, it's green yellow orange etc, lots of brush and grass. We start up. Single file at first. I keep my steady solid pace trying to get my body warmed up. I am staying so positive and confident. I've trained for this, I am conditioned, I am ready. Anything the trainers quiz me on I answer confidently. I can learn procedures quickly. We stop at times to do hd, fk, burpees, push ups, bicycles, and cut line, then get back to hike. I feel good, strong, tired, but I know I can do this all day. I've trained for this, I am conditioned, focused, solidly stacked. I keep saying this in my head. I am doing this. We are all here together. I am ready. I continue to push at my strong steady pace with the QB on my shoulder. I switch off time to time to give each shoulder a rest, never stopping my forward momentum. We keep pushing. I am not far behind, in fact I'm with a group of rookies, not by myself. We push together. We got this.”

Notice the use of colors, textures, and emotions in her visualization. She even practices her mantra in her head, and she strategizes how she will handle the weight of the QB. The literature on visualization suggests that adding detail from all five senses strengthens the effects of imagery. However, what I loved most is that she ended her imagery with teamwork. That is ultimately what helps rookies through the rigors of smokejumper preparation—a reliance and dedication to the team. If a physically talented but self-serving rookie shows up to rookie training, they won't last a week. This process is not just about being a physical specimen. Rookies must also show their dedication to the team. The purpose of rookie training is to physically test incoming rookies to ensure their bodies and minds can withstand the job demands, all while mentally and psychologically preparing them for the job of smokejumping. Entailed in the psychological prep is the glaring necessity of teamwork. Teamwork helps smokejumpers stay alive and well through the dangerous and demanding work they perform.

MONDAY, MARCH 20, 2017 (4 WEEKS OUT)

This week, Jess and I explored San Francisco to see if we wanted to move there after Redlands. I took a week off at the gym, and Jess was on spring break from her classes at Loma Linda. We took two days to drive up, taking our time along the Pacific Coast Highway. The weather changed often over the 400-mile journey from rainy, cloudy, and cold to hot, humid, and sunny. It was a "super-bloom" year in Southern California, meaning it rained a lot during winter, and the wildflowers painted the freeway hillsides in giant seas of rich yellow and orange pastels.

When we finally arrived in San Francisco, we underwent the full tourist experience, hiking down and up the hills of Chinatown and the San Francisco stairs, riding the trolley, visiting the wax museum, exploring the wharf, hiking Muir Woods, and eating lunch in Sausalito. I felt so free. It was my first week-long break from coaching and the master's program in a long time. That didn't mean I took a break from Heidi, though. She was at her most crucial junction where volume and intensity are both high. I made sure to check on Heidi throughout the week and brought my laptop just in case she needed last-minute programming changes.

After five months of training, we had finally arrived at this very moment. The peak week! The edge. The most dangerous and potentially fruitful segment of Heidi's preparation. This week was loaded with the highest volumes of running, hiking, and PT. I had scheduled more than 20 training hours spread over six days:

Monday (5 hours): Imagery, full warm-up, running intervals, and a four-hour hike with 60 pounds at elevation through the forest, with exercises, cooldown and foot care and recovery afterwards

Tuesday (4.5 hours): Imagery, full warm-up, Hill sprints, 7 rounds of high volume PT, 6-mile easy run, hip and core stability work, swimming, and yoga, cooldown, and foot care and recovery afterwards

Wednesday (2.5 hours): Imagery, full warm-up, heavy pack training, strength and power training, cooldown, and foot care and recovery afterwards

Thursday (3.5 hours): Imagery, full warm-up, PT density training, a lower body strength metcon and an upper body stability sequence, intervals, yoga, and swimming, cooldown, and foot care and recovery afterwards

Friday (2.5 hours): Imagery, full warm-up, intervals, a 75-pound hike for an hour and a half, and ended with hip and core stability, cooldown, and foot care and recovery afterwards

Saturday (3.5 hours): Imagery, full warm-up, a half-marathon competition trail run, and ended with some easy-paced full body stability, cooldown, and foot care and recovery afterwards

She completely crushed Monday, but we did have a little scare. When I read her spreadsheets, I thought that her season was over before it started. On her hike, she wrote, "Just had quite a scare on the way down! Stepped on a snake both of us doing the hot coal dance OMG! Part of the job but always takes my breath away and thank god it wasn't a rattlesnake. Good on Cali's (calisthenics)." I responded: "LOL this is scary!! Yes thank god no rattler!!! Jess and I were hiking in Muir Woods yesterday and she stepped on a little garder snake."

We played with some strict pull-up drop sets this week to stimulate lactate, and Heidi squeezed out three extra reps, a 10% increase. I hoped this stimulus would help her push the pull-ups in the rookie training PT test to another large personal best.

To end this brutal training week, on Saturday Heidi competed in a half-marathon trail run and took first place for the females. She then sat in a car for 4 hours as she drove to Vegas. She was headed to Boise tomorrow! We got through peak week without an injury! Now, onto the taper. I hoped that all of Heidi's physical capacities would gel over the next three weeks before day one.

I had been thoroughly wrapped up in my own life, and Jess in hers. We rarely had time for each other. The spring break San Francisco trip was exactly what we needed to slow down and reconnect. On our last vacation night, Jess and I walked to a French restaurant for dinner. As we ate foods that we'd never heard of before and haven't eaten since, I drank an old-fashioned, and Jess downed a few glasses of cabernet. She snarked dry jokes that were still hard for me to decipher as jokes, even after being together six years. We talked about our future. Jess was going into a clinical lab science program, and I had a few more months left working on my master's. She wondered if I would ever give myself a day off from work. I laughed and said, "What about this week?" I could tell that she was serious. I countered, asking when she would take a day off from studying. She said it wasn't the same thing. To lighten the mood, she poked fun at my first gray hairs which had recently begun to sprout out of my temples. She joked that I would be completely gray by 40 if I kept this pace up. At least I could make time to take her out for a nice French dinner, I retorted. I also assured her that I was almost done with programming for Heidi.

Later that night, I wondered if Jess was jealous of the women I trained. I hoped not. Was I pushing too hard? Full-time coaching at the gym, evenings and Saturdays for master's work, and Sunday, a full day sitting at the kitchen table, programming. Now that Jess had pointed it out, I thought I would like a day off sometime in the future. I hoped my efforts would all be worth it one day. Perhaps Heidi would make it through after all. Who knew what that would lead to?

MONDAY, MARCH 27, 2017 (3 WEEKS OUT)

We had done it. We made it through the apex week and were onto Heidi's first week of tapering. I dropped her training duration down to 15 hours and began to increase the intensity. Now that training volume was decreasing, I could increase Heidi's running speed. Even though many injuries are volume related, and we were decreasing volume, when the intensity ticks up while the volume is still relatively high, bad things can happen. I made sure to detail every ounce of Heidi's training to minimize risk.

Over the weekend, Heidi had made the drive to Boise and was now training there. She planned to catch some training sessions with her "rookie bro's and sisters." I programmed one more week of PT lactate training for her pull-ups, push-ups, and sit-ups. She squeezed out one extra pull-up this week, a good sign that she had completed enough lactate training and it was now time to start decreasing both the volume and intensity of her training. We had gotten all we could over the past five months. Now it was time to reveal what we had created.

After all this time working towards the heavy pack test, this week we moved the pack weight up to 110 pounds. The test weight! She wrote, "3x1 miles, 110 lbs., in 15:56, 16:28, 17:21 ... WHAT!?!? Sweeet!!! Felt good. 110 lbs. !!!" This warmed my heart. The week after her heaviest volume training, Heidi had crushed her heaviest carry yet, just ten pounds below her bodyweight, and finished in just over 55 minutes. Finally, Heidi passing the heavy pack test became vividly real. We were right there.

For the light pack hike this week, I took her down from 60 pounds to 50 and dropped her training time to two hours. For PT, she completed six rounds of high-volume pull-ups, push-ups, and sit-ups with a small decrease in the reps compared to the previous week. In her sprint session, Heidi ran with some of the other rookies who had also arrived in Boise. She wrote, "Ran in blizzard rain! With 3 other rookies. So much fun. They pushed me. But I was right there with them!!! Not always last either ;)"

At the end of the week, Heidi completed a hike with 8 of the guys from her rookie cohort. She wrote, "75 lbs. at lucky peak good steep shorter hike, 30min up, calisthenics then 30min down finished with calisthenics at the car. We hiked with 8 of the rookies and I was last and maybe 3min behind but I kept my pace, I can only go my pace. I feel good, muscles a little tight and sore but feeling good. Beautiful weather today. Total distance 2miles." She was behind but kept up. I hoped that we had done enough. I also reminded myself that she was coming off a monster training week and would be fatigued for another week or two before she began to reveal her true potential.

When she made it through the week and felt ok with no nagging issues, I felt a wave of relief. Whew! We made it this far, only two more weeks to go. Home stretch. We weren't out of the woods just yet, but the light was now visible on the horizon.

MONDAY, APRIL 3, 2017 (2 WEEKS OUT)

Heidi had been in Boise for a week. She was acclimating to Boise's elevation and weather and getting to know her fellow rookies. Monday April 3, 2017, Heidi was scheduled to complete her final PT test before heading into rookie training in two weeks. Going into this week, I was under the impression that the rookie trainers told Heidi she could take a practice run at the pack test after the PT test, and that she could pick whatever weight she wanted. Because it was just practice. At least that's what she told me, so I planned one last heavy pack training session for her later in the week.

That morning, I felt my phone vibrate and saw Heidi calling. Any unexpected call from Heidi immediately shot my adrenaline up a few notches. I took a breath, let it out slowly, and calmed myself. I arched an eyebrow and shook my head, surprised. When she called, it would be on the weekends. At first, I was concerned that she had injured something while training in Boise. I felt that familiar and uncomfortable jolt of anxiety in my stomach. My inner thoughts reminded me not to jump to conclusions, see what she needs. It's a coach's worst nightmare to have an athlete tweak an ankle with the final competition so close at hand! When I answered, I could tell immediately that something good had happened. Heidi exclaimed that she had passed her pack test!

Confused, I asked what she meant. "You were scheduled to do a practice round this week with your rookie trainers, right?" She replied yes, but this morning, they said she could get the test over with if she wanted, and she chose that route. And she nailed it! 110 pounds (she only weighed 120 at the time of the test) for three miles on a flat course, completed in 50:37, setting a personal best time for this test by about 25 minutes. Her previous best time was 75 minutes and that took a lot out of her. It also washed her out of rookie training last year on the first day. This time around, she finished much faster and felt great!

The last six months of progressing steadily from 30 pounds all the way up to 110 pounds in training paid off handsomely. I was very proud of her. This was a momentum-building event heading into rookie training in a week and a half. She now knew that she was physically lightyears beyond last year. If this was any indication on how rookie training would go, then Heidi was in for some impressive performances.

During this week, she also performed another PT test. Her scores weren't her best, but they were very close: 19 pull-ups, 89 push-ups, 139 sit-ups, and the 1.5-mile in 9:15, into a headwind! I was expecting her to beat her PRs from last month and was stumped as to why she hadn't. Then I realized the reason. She was still fatigued from the training volume peak two weeks ago. The taper was still taking place, and her body was not yet fully recovered.

Even though she still had some recovering left to do, I believed the taper was working well, maybe even better than I had hoped. At the end of this second taper week, Heidi felt noticeably good. Her shin pain was almost gone, and her feet felt ok. Her body was healing itself because the workload decreased further each week. With the psychologically weighty heavy pack training checked off the to-do list, now she could relax a touch. She conquered that massive dragon, but there was still one scaley, bitter, fire-breathing beast remaining—the jump tower.

MONDAY, APRIL 10, 2017 (1 WEEK OUT)

During the final week of training, Heidi completed six hours of light training. Compared to her peak week, this was about one quarter of the total work time and less than 25% of the volume. Her soreness and fatigue dissipated further, but not all the way. And she trained alone. The rest of the rookies took the week off to recover. I wrote her what I thought would be some easy hiking and intervals. A few more pull-ups, push-ups, and sit-ups. At the end of the week, I saw some worrying feedback. She wrote, "I'm feeling like a broken spring, broken & rusty. A little emotional at the end of sprints. Just frustrated. They were more like striders than sprints. Quads feel sore. Getting a massage tomorrow." My heart sank. I thought this low volume training week would put a nicely wrapped bow on her preparation. We had done too much this week. I immediately felt a sensation of pressure in my chest. I felt like I had let her down and began to worry.

That weekend I was sweating bullets in my hot apartment, pacing back and forth as the psychological weight of this week sat heavy on my shoulders. Had we done enough work over the last five and a half months? Had we pushed her far enough? Had we left any gains on the table? Had we tapered enough? Had she recovered? After her last note in the training sheets, it seemed like she was still physically banged up. My ideal taper would have left her feeling zero soreness, completely fresh, healed, and ready.

Would she go into rookie training flat that first week and quit? No, she'd rather die than quit. What if she didn't make it this time after putting in all these hard days, weeks, and months of work? Money spent? All that time at my stupid kitchen table pretending that I knew what I was doing, deep down knowing that it was a crapshoot at best. What if she failed and told people that I had failed her? She did a marvelous job of doing exactly what was written, so it would be on me if we did too much. What if she got injured and sued me? I continued to catastrophize, a bad habit that I had learned in high school while going through bouts of anxiety driven by hormones run amok. I did not tell Heidi any of this, of course. Best battle your own demons in your head. Outwardly, I pretended that I was confident. There was no time left to add any more wood to the fire, or to take any away. She was headed into rookie training with exactly what she had. Soon we'd see if it was enough.

Up in Boise, alone with her thoughts, I'm sure Heidi was more nervous than I was, and it was very unpleasant for me. I can be a pain in the ass when I'm stressed, and I was short with Jess, who shrugged it off and made fun of me, which made me even angrier.

I woke up on Saturday night in a puddle of my own sweat after a stress dream about waiting tables where I showed up late to my job and had tables continuing to walk in, and the restaurant ran out of ranch dressing, and I dropped two pizzas on the ground and lost everyone's checks.

On Sunday, I went for a hike up in Forest Falls on Heidi's favorite trail. The whole day felt hollow. I didn't program at the table. There was no more programming to write. The time had come. Tomorrow, Heidi would begin.

MONDAY, APRIL 17, 2017 (FIRST WEEK OF ROOKIE TRAINING)

Heidi's first week of rookie training came and went. I had been used to multiple texts throughout the week and an occasional phone call and logging into Google spreadsheets to check for her detailed, upbeat, and entertaining feedback on our live training spreadsheet. This week, crickets. The silence was deafening. I had extra time now that Heidi's programming hours were off my plate, so I went for a swim in the apartment pool and recited my own mantra: *I speak the truth, I don't take things personally, I don't assume, and I do my best.* I was hoping with all my might that Heidi was doing her best. She knew no other way.

I didn't hear from Heidi until Saturday. She called me. She sounded tired, excited. She had made it through the first week! She had set personal bests for everything, including the pack test! She had shaved off another 3 or 4 minutes, completing that 110 lb. 3-mile carry in sub-16-minute miles at a bodyweight of 125 lbs. Amazing. I sighed and smiled, shaking my head. A small amount of pressure released from my chest. I told her I was proud of her. Go get it next week. There was a long way yet, and anything could happen.

She informed me that after the severe physical beatdown they had all experienced that week, a handful of her fellow rookies had washed out. One washout was the other female. Heidi was now the sole woman. There were now nine rookies left. Despite being by far the smallest rookie, Heidi was holding her own on the hikes, running, and PT. She was sore and exhausted, but she had been through this before.

MONDAY, APRIL 24, 2017 (SECOND WEEK OF ROOKIE TRAINING)

No word from Heidi during the second week. I texted her on Friday night asking how the week went. She wrote back that she had made it through, more physically beat up, fatigued. Her shins felt sore, but her foot was ok for now. Overall, she was holding her own. A couple more rookies had washed this week. Down to seven.

I drove up to Cedar City, Utah to graduate from Southern Utah University. I left at 6 a.m. to arrive in time for the event at noon. I drove alone because Jess was finishing up her clinical rounds at the hospital. After cruising along in the car for an hour with six to go, I noticed how much I enjoyed driving. Sitting still. Not doing anything. Breathing. I began to time my breaths with the mile markers and attempted to cycle one long slow full breath each mile. I felt deflated, dried out. Chewed up. The past few months had been insane with work, school, and Heidi. Now that was all coming to an end. I hoped Heidi had what it took. We had both been through a lot.

During the graduation, I was designated Student of the Year for the Sport Conditioning and Performance Master of Science Program. They attributed the award to my thesis defense on collegiate female rugby athletes. All that preparation for my presentation had paid off. I hoped the many hours over the past half year preparing Heidi would pay off as well.

After the graduation, I caught a late lunch at my favorite BBQ place in Cedar City and drove the 7 hours back home again. No time to stay the night. I had programming to do tomorrow for a handful of athletes.

MONDAY, MAY 1, 2017 (THIRD WEEK OF ROOKIE TRAINING)

During Heidi's third week after the severe physical beatdown of weeks one and two, I was expecting her to start experiencing the extreme soreness and fatigue that can set in after training nonstop at high volume for a few weeks at elevation as she competed against men ten years younger. At the end of the week, I received an excited phone call from Heidi. She'd made it through the week, and she had performed better than ever—during rookie training, while sore, tired, and fatigued. This was a total slam dunk for Heidi, and for me! My periodization strategy had worked. In theory, if stress (the peak month) and then recovery (the taper) are maximized, an athlete or team will physically peak their performance for 1 to 3 weeks depending on the duration of the training cycle leading up to the competitive period. Heidi was performing better than ever in the middle of rookie training. I really couldn't believe it. I had predicted and hoped beforehand the taper would allow her to feel fresh and would peak her for the second and maybe the third week, but I had never done this with an athlete. I was ecstatic at her results. This is when I first believed that what we had done was special. It was at this point that I knew the only thing that could stop her now was the jump tower. This is what crushed Heidi's dream in her first year at rookie training in McCall. It was time for redemption.

MONDAY, MAY 8, 2017 (FOURTH WEEK OF ROOKIE TRAINING)

This week was a blur for me. I felt helpless waiting to hear back from Heidi. I checked my phone constantly for a mid-week text. Or worse, a call. If she contacted me mid-week, that might signify the end of her dream.

On Saturday, Heidi texted me that she had made it through the week. She was too exhausted to call. Not much to tell, either. She was having some trouble learning the jump commands. The jump tower was challenging. Her legs were constantly sore. Her shins were yelling at her. She began to feel her foot pain again. I thought back to the thousands of step-ups and training hours and miles spent hiking with a heavy pack for those long training hikes. Six months of madness. I felt small, helpless. There was nothing I could do to help. All I could do was wait for her call.

MONDAY, MAY 15, 2017 (FIFTH WEEK OF ROOKIE TRAINING)

My phone pocket was burning on my right hip. I received hundreds of phantom texts that week. I'd look at my phone after feeling a vibration. Nothing. No text. Was I going crazy? Finally, sweet relief. Heidi texted on the weekend simply that she'd made it through another week. I asked her how it had gone, and she said that she was still in, and things were ok. She was still practicing her jump commands and PLFs. Her body was in a constant state of soreness and fatigue. I asked when they would be done, and she said that she didn't know. For her, it was one foot in front of the other, full speed. For me, more waiting. Heidi mentioned that she and her rookie brothers were told by the rookie trainers that they were never doing enough. They weren't working hard enough. They weren't going to cut it. This, of course, was the rookie trainers mushing the group towards the edge, pushing them as far as they could.

MONDAY, MAY 22, 2017 (SIXTH WEEK OF ROOKIE TRAINING)

While Heidi was away at rookie training, I simply stuck my head in the sand and waited, not knowing how long it would take. She said somewhere around 4–7 weeks. The longest she had made it in the past was halfway through week four. We had just passed week five, and she was still in. Barely, it felt. I played the waiting game and passed the time coaching personal training sessions and group classes at the CrossFit gym, working with my rugby team, coaching Emily at the strongman gym, training hard myself, and reciting my mantra before diving into the pool. Even Jess didn't have much time for me right now. She was nose-deep into her clinical hours, and her schedule was changing every two weeks. Mornings. Afternoons. Noc-shifts. I wondered what it would be like for Heidi right now, what she would be doing. Physically suffering through long runs, rucking, endless PT. Climbing the jump tower, practicing parachute lands. Taking actual practice jumps out of a plane. Acting as a team player.

In the middle of week six, I felt a vibration on my right hip. A call from Heidi! I got a sick feeling in my stomach. My catastrophizing mind spun out of control in a moment's time as I moved my finger to accept the call. Had she broken an ankle on a bad parachute landing? Had they washed her because she had failed the jump protocols one too many times? While Heidi was undergoing training for the previous six months, I must have kept my nose so close to the grindstone that I had barely given myself time to look up and see how deep into Heidi's journey I had fallen. I was in all the way. I hoped with all my being that she was successful.

I summoned the courage and answered the phone. "Heidi?" I said. She chimed in her high-pitched voice, "Fritz, I made it!" Sweet relief washed over me as I stood in the center of the gym. I had been distracting myself with a grueling training session of snatches, box jumps, and sprinting, my favorite combination. I yelled out a loud whoop!!! I jumped up, landed, rolled onto my back, still clutching the phone against my ear. My heart pounded in my chest. My smile spread from ear to ear. I kicked my feet against the ground as I laughed with Heidi. She was laughing, too! I could sense her excitement, her relief. She sounded invigorated despite her extreme fatigue. Heidi then went off about the past few days and what she and the other remaining rookies had gone through. She couldn't believe it. She thanked me profusely and said that she couldn't have done it without me. I congratulated her and thanked her for trusting me.

A month passed by. Things slowed down. After taking what felt like a giant deep breath in my life, I looked back at what had happened during my journey coaching Heidi over the last half a year. I was living week by week, day by day sometimes. My fitness had suffered. I didn't know which way was up. Some weekends, I had spent upwards of eight hours each Sunday programming for Heidi and a few other athletes, and it seemed unsustainable. Jess and I had not spent much quality time together despite our upcoming union next spring. To top it all off, I had a lingering feeling that Heidi's success was pure luck. And it felt like there was no one I could share my experience with. My colleagues at the gym didn't have the patience to sit down and sift through thirty tabs on a spreadsheet, each 100 lines or more, to decipher and give their opinion on what we had done. The closest I came to professional closure on my performance with coaching Heidi was a conversation with Mike, who was finishing up his 2017 track and field season and preparing his remaining jumpers for the national championships. Funny enough, when he had worked at Redlands, Heidi was one of his distance athletes in the first years of his coaching career. He thought what Heidi and I had done was impressive. I was just grateful that Heidi had shown up to rookie training, crushed it, and now she was able to live her dream. She had become a smokejumper.

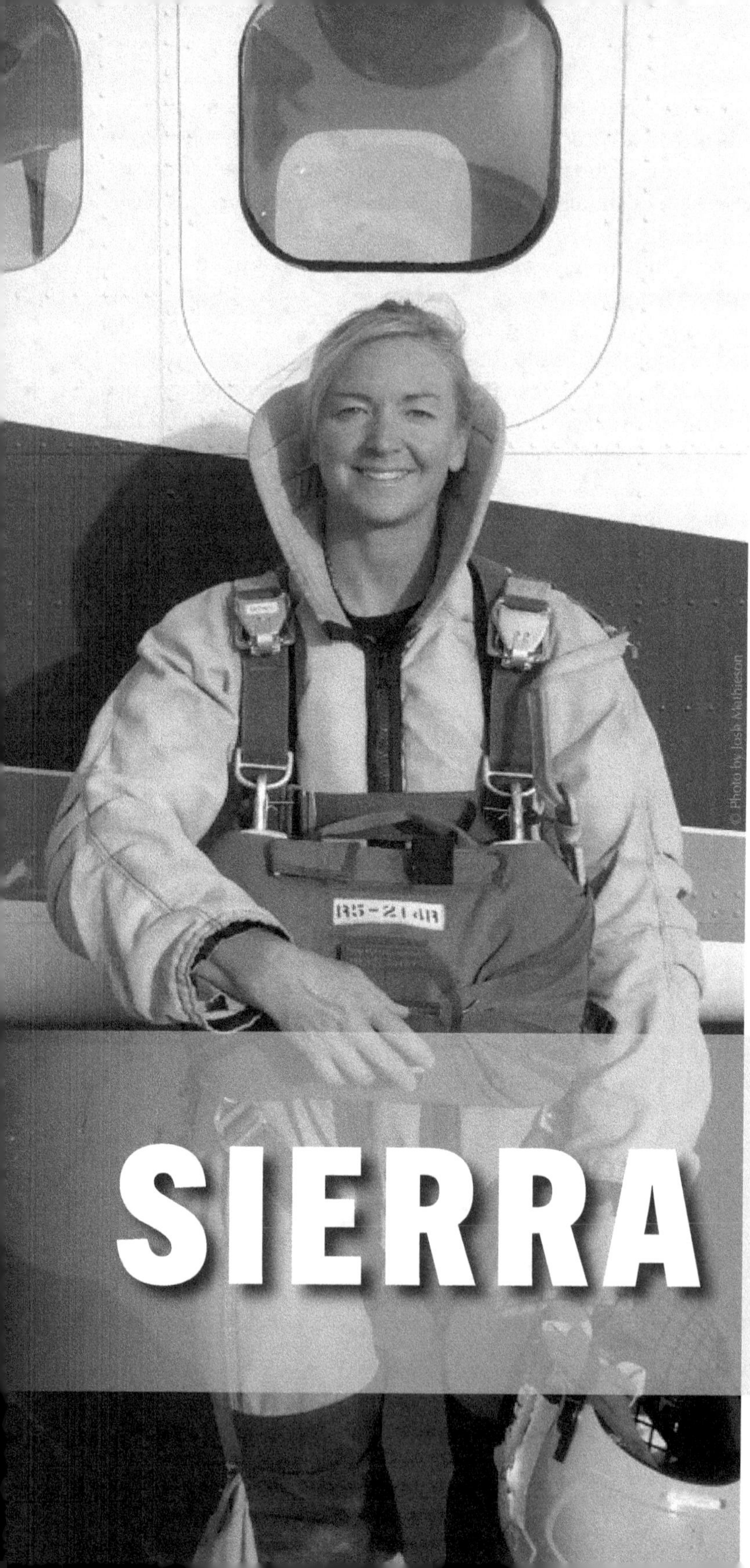

© Photo by Josh Mathieson

3

SIERRA

HEIDI BECAME A SMOKEJUMPER, AND WORD SPREAD. Female smokejumpers are rare, especially at the Bureau of Land Management smokejumper bases due to the extreme physical demands of rookie training. Heidi was known in the world of wildland fire before she made it through smokejumper selection, and she crushed it. A 5'2," 120 pound, 35-year-old female completed rookie training at Boise. How did she do it? Other female wildland firefighters who saw themselves as potential smokejumpers became interested in learning her secret. Even the media wanted to hear and share the story of Heidi's success! When a female becomes a smokejumper, it's big news.

Other females contacted Heidi to ask about her experience. She told them about her three years of experience at smokejumper rookie training, and she would mention how big of an impact working with me had on her success that third season. From Heidi's networking, I received a handful of referrals at the end of the 2017 wildfire season.

Once Heidi made a connection with a woman in fire who was interested in chatting with me, it was my job to hop on a phone call with them. In the off-season of October 2017, I talked to a couple of women, but none of them seemed like they were dead set on becoming smokejumpers or on paying me, some wildland fire outsider, to help them train. I think some of the women didn't understand how I could help them since I had zero experience as a firefighter myself, specifically wildland fire, and very little firefighter coaching experience other than Heidi. I had coached a few city firefighters at the CrossFit gym in Redlands, but I didn't write them specific training. Athlete recruitment is a numbers game, and eventually I got lucky and found my next candidate.

One day, Heidi mentioned a new potential smokejumper who was interested in speaking with me. Heidi said she was an older woman (and Heidi was very old as far as smokejumpers go, especially females) who she knew from the Del Rosa Hotshots. Her age already intrigued me. Heidi had passed along my information, saying she might give me a call to pick my brain on how to train for smokejumper rookie training. I told Heidi that I was willing to help as much as I could. I'm not sure how well Heidi and this other woman got along, but I assume they had a passable relationship. The new woman trusted Heidi's recommendation enough to get in contact with me. From what Heidi had heard, this woman was seriously interested in attempting smokejumper rookie training. Then a few weeks went by without a phone call, and I forgot all about her.

Within the past six months, Jess and I found ourselves swept up by a whirlwind of change. Earlier in the year, I had graduated from Southern Utah University with my Master of Science degree in Sport Conditioning and Performance. This left me feeling even more confident in my coaching ability, especially after winning the Student of the Year award. A few months later, Jess had graduated from Loma Linda University with a bachelor's degree (her second bachelor's) in Clinical Lab Science (CLS). Within two months after graduating, Jessica sought out a CLS position at Kaiser in San Diego and, with no experience other than her clinical rounds, landed a job! She had accomplished exactly what she had set out to do three years earlier. I had to hold up my end of the bargain, so we finalized our decision to move to San Diego.

A few weeks had passed since my last chat with Heidi, and I was wrapped up in the events of my own life. It was the middle of October, and I was planning our move down to San Diego. For the first month of Jessica's employment in San Diego, she was commuting about 90–120 minutes one-way to work in San Diego from our place in Redlands. We didn't see each other much. I was finishing up coaching my in-person clients in Redlands and saying goodbye to my friends. Our lease was up in a week, so we were packing boxes in our tiny apartment when I received a call from an unknown number.

It was Heidi's smokejumper hopeful colleague. An awkward phone call ensued. We had not met before, and I was distracted by the clutter and chaos generated from the boxes and furniture lying all over the place. From the beginning, I got a sense that I had to prove myself to her. She seemed unsure whether I would be able to help her. I also got the feeling that she expected me to have more experience coaching firefighters than I did. I was honest with her and said that Heidi was my entire resume. The conversation was clunky. After Heidi's success, I thought that I'd earned some respect, but now it felt like an illusion. And probably for the best, too. Overconfidence has always led me to a necessary lesson in humility.

This new woman was immediately a conundrum. She spoke in fire jargon which brought back memories of my very first conversation with Heidi, and I cracked a smile. This time around, I followed her story a little more clearly. She displayed the same special forces cadence in her voice, a mixture of frankness, calmness, and stoicism. After this initial call, I thought that she wasn't too serious. She wanted to continue to work as a full-time firefighter as she trained for smokejumper rookie training. To me, this didn't make sense. From my limited understanding after working with Heidi, anyone who wanted to pass rookie training would have to train full time like Heidi. How could anyone train as much as Heidi while also working full time?! This woman said that she was overweight from drinking too much wine and eating too much food, and when I asked where she lived, she laughed and said it was complicated. In addition, she was almost 40 years old. At this point, I became confused and wondered what she thought she was doing chasing smokejumping at all. By now, I knew they didn't let just anyone "try out." Candidates had years of wildland firefighting under their belt and leadership experience. While she did have years of experience, I found out that she did not yet have a candidate offer from a smokejumper base. She was actively seeking.

During the next part of our conversation, my eyes steadily grew wider until my eyebrows were up against my hairline, furrowing my brow. She was an endurance athlete and ran ultramarathons. Whew. That brought me some relief.

If you want to be a smokejumper, you must have some specific and dominant physical skill that you can rely on to help get you through. I think Heidi's was stubbornness mixed with relentless desire.

Anyone that can go out and run 50 to 100-plus mile races indicates their structure and endurance must be sound. I thought this to myself during the call. However, I was still torn by the combination of her daily drinking, being overweight by her standards (if I had to guess, probably about 10 pounds over her competitive ultrarunner bodyweight, not clinically overweight), and wanting to continue working full time instead of taking time off from work to train full time. It seemed like she thought she could train a little bit and be fine. After what I had witnessed Heidi go through, I had a feeling that no one can do the bare minimum and pass rookie training. They make you earn every single inch.

After this initial conversation, I reflected on my first impressions and jotted my feelings down in my training notebook below the other information that I had taken down during our call. She seemed laissez-faire about the whole situation, and she didn't seem too sold on my coaching ability. I was ok with that. I guess I had to prove myself to her.

When challenged by an athlete, it brings out some deep-rooted self-doubt. I have always lacked complete belief in my abilities, even when I had sound outcomes to show for my efforts. In Heidi's case, I left room for the chance that her success was a fluke. Perhaps she had succeeded despite my efforts to help her. That was still a possibility. With this new woman, I might have also been afraid to be vulnerable with someone whom I had just met. With Heidi, I knew her beforehand, and within the first week of coaching her, she had let me into her bubble, and I had let her within mine. Maybe I was afraid to let this new athlete into my space because I didn't yet know her. Either way, she had decided to proceed with me. Her name was Sierra.

In the following days, I began to question my desire to attempt preparing another candidate for rookie training. Even though Sierra wanted to train with me, did I have the bandwidth to take her on? Could I handle another smokejumper?

During the past year while coaching Heidi, I had spent hours every Sunday for six months straight sitting at my kitchen table, drafting, and creating her programming each week. It weighed on my wellness, and it took a toll on my relationship with Jess, who constantly complained that I work too much and didn't take any days off. It was true. I would work Monday through Friday, film videos in my free time on Saturday, and would spend half the day on Sunday creating the week's programming for my group of online training athletes. Mid-week at home between coaching shifts, I went into the spreadsheets to track Heidi's progress and adjust volumes based on her feedback. I was obsessed. Could I do all that again? Was the potential success of coaching two women to become smokejumpers worth the price that I had to pay?

My negativity spiraled further downwards. Everything in my life right now was about to change. I was moving from Redlands—a place that I enjoyed, a place where my college friends lived, a small town where I was known. At the grocery store, I'd run into members from the gym, and I knew the clerks. I felt good here. Comfortable. San Diego was brand new. Uncomfortable. It felt cold, distant. There, I knew no one. Was no one. I had no job waiting for me. I had a nagging fear that I would lose myself in the city. Many years ago, I had chosen Redlands for college instead of ASU in Tempe because the small town of Redlands had a warmer draw for me.

After letting my amygdala run amok for some time, I realized these thoughts were unhealthy. Whenever I begin to spiral downwards, getting out in nature, alone, was helpful. Even though I had plenty of packing left to do, I drove up to Forest Falls for one last push up my favorite hike, the Momyer Creek Trail to Dobbs Cabin, a route that Heidi also loved. My preferred entrance to this hike was on private property. I am partial to this entrance even though there is another public trailhead further up the road because it's the steepest start to any trail I've ever seen, so after being turned away before by the church that owns the land, now after parking my car on the side of the road a quarter mile away, I ran with my pack, booking it to the trailhead and up the hill a few hundred feet as a golf cart pulled up below, a man yelling at me "HEY! YOU'RE ON PRIVATE PROPERTY AND YOU NEED TO LEAVE!!!" I stopped and turned around to take a look at the big guy in the cart and realized he wasn't going to set foot up this trail to come after me and slowed to a walk. Jess also gets a thrill outrunning the golf cart surveillance, but today she was down in San Diego working at the hospital.

The trail was so steep, it burned my legs, calves, and lungs. The trail begins with over two thousand feet of elevation gain in the first three miles. In other words, it's steep as hell, and sucks the wind right out of you, plus it starts at 5300 feet. It's lovely. While hiking, I imagined Heidi hiking this very trail the year before, pushing faster than I was now, and in the snow, while carrying sixty pounds on her back. Crazy. I hoped that Sierra would be as pleasant of an experience to work with as Heidi.

This would be my final time hiking Momyer. By the end of my forest bathing, my head had cleared. I realized that coaching Sierra was an awesome opportunity to help prepare another woman to test herself at smokejumper rookie training, and I decided to take her on. I also realized this was an opportunity to test myself as well. Was Heidi a fluke? Could I help another female through? It would have to be a team effort. If I failed to prepare Sierra well, she'd surely fail. And if I did my job and she failed to show up at full mental and psychological capacity, then we would both fail as well. For the moment, I pushed my doubts down deep, deciding subconsciously to deal with them some other time.

On the hike, I also thought about my imminent future. The move to San Diego seemed both daunting and ripe with potential. Jess was making enough to support both of us for now, so I could tinker and craft a new pathway. I would have some income from a handful of my current Redlands clients who wanted to begin remote coaching after the move. On top of all the change, Jess and I had a wedding date set for May 2018, a few weeks into Sierra's hypothetical smokejumper rookie training start date! It was going to be a big year.

Heidi was my first and only wildland firefighter, so she was my sole reference point for expectations. So far, Sierra was an anomaly. Right from the beginning, the differences between the two women were striking. Sierra liked to party. She drank beer and wine most nights. She liked to eat well and dined with friends and family often. She was also an incredible distance athlete. She ran many ultra-endurance events, won a few, and placed near the top in others. She could go out on the weekend and run further in a single day than I would ask Heidi run in an entire week. It was surprisingly difficult to wrap my head around the type of athlete Sierra was. I had to rid myself of the notion that I would be training Heidi again. Sierra was not Heidi, and their personalities, athletic ability, and approach to the world were vastly different. With these differences came a large dose of learning on my part. Sierra seemed extreme and a bit cocksure, almost brash, yet humble enough to admit that she had gotten by in the past simply by showing up and coasting on her talent alone. That approach ended this season. It had to. No one coasts through smokejumper rookie training.

Our coaching relationship was not easy on Sierra, either. The door swung both ways. She had to learn to deal with me, too. I thrived through structure. I lived in the spreadsheets, comforted by the data and energized by the predictability. Sierra was the opposite. She lived deep below the surface of the gulf of California off the Baja Peninsula with a spear gun in her hand, hunting massive fish. She seemed to seek life twenty miles into a run up and down a steep and narrow mountain trail. She seemed to live everywhere. Full of life, and her life was full. I soon found out that she literally did live... everywhere.

> Many athletes make use of the positive training adaptations from living at high altitude. The saying goes, "live high, train low", which means live at altitude and train at lower elevations. In Southern California, this is logistically possible. Forest Falls is about a mile high and less than 30-minute drive from Redlands, whose elevation is slightly above 1000 feet. Heidi would make use of this beneficial geographical advantage, completing her endurance training at elevation in Forest Falls and her speed training down on the University of Redlands track.

Sierra had a ton of places that she slept. She currently worked as a San Diego structural firefighter, which was a very challenging position for her to land. When she wasn't sleeping at the station on shift, she had a boat in a slip in some bay in Mexico. Yep, she lived on a boat. In another country. She lived on two boats, actually. When she wasn't in Mexico on her own boat, she could also stay on her dad's boat in the Coronado Marina. Furthermore, she was in the process of building a house in Mexico, from scratch. She boasted of building an entire wall made from wine bottles that she drank! In addition to the fire station and two boats, she also spent time living and training at a cabin that she owned up in Forest Falls, not too far away from Heidi's cabin. She could train at altitude and in the snow, which make for good and challenging training. To say that logistics would be an issue in preparing Sierra for smokejumper rookie training is a drastic understatement. Right about then, I felt wholly overwhelmed.

When training Heidi, she was a full-time athlete. I could write her 3 to 5 hours of training a day and she had no excuses. She'd complete exactly what I had written for her on the day that it was designated to be accomplished. Sierra, on the other hand, was a full-time firefighter in San Diego. Her schedule was standard as far as firefighters go. She'd work a handful of days in a row, sometimes a week or more, followed by long stretches of time off. This threw a wrench into my linear and predictable weekly plan that had worked so well for Heidi.

There was one silver lining in Sierra's work situation—firefighters are allowed to dedicate time while on shift to PT. The caveat here is the workouts had to be short, just in case a call came in. I couldn't send her on long hikes, bike rides, swims, or runs while on shift. Those would have to wait until she was off. To further complicate things, when she had a few days in a row off work, she took vacations or road trips. The logistics of planning Sierra's program was becoming my worst nightmare.

And if things couldn't get any more complicated, Sierra was also smack-dab in the middle of a master's program, her second master's, to be exact. I was wondering how on earth she planned to complete all these things each week. The full-time physically demanding job, the master's program, and the many hours of smokejumper preparation.

To help myself initially plan for Sierra's multiple living situations, I created a graphic containing each living situation and the specific training opportunities each provided:

Forest Falls Training Opportunities	*SD Firehouse Training Opportunities*	*Mexico / Boat Training Opportunities*	*Dad's Coronado Marina Training Opportunities*
Mountains (hiking)	Bumper plates & bars	Hiking trails	Small gym
LA Fitness	Kettlebells	A long flat beach	Dumbbells
Yoga	Pull-up bar	Ocean (swimming)	Cardio machines
Crafton hills pool	Dumbbells	** 50 lb weight vest	Pull-up bar
Mountain bike	Rowing machine		Road bike
Doorway pull-up bar	Bike		Beach: surf, run
** 50 lb weight vest	Treadmill		** 50 lb weight vest
	Dirt road		
	Ultimate frisbee		
	** 50 lb weight vest		

Each of the four situations had their own pros and cons. We couldn't train every aspect of what was necessary for Sierra to prepare in any one week's time. Instead, we'd have to piece things together as best we could. Some weeks there would be hiking opportunities with minimal strength training. Other weeks would be training at the firehouse with no running or hiking for many days in a row. I could foresee this was the biggest limitation to my planning process. At least that was my assessment before we started training together. Then things became even more complicated.

Besides the complexity of programming multiple capacities of strength and conditioning and relying on multiple locations with vastly different training modalities at each, I wanted to better assess Sierra's physical strengths and limitations. I am a big fan of spending some time each week bolstering my athlete's strengths, not just improving their weaknesses. After a fire season where fire athlete physical capacities are decreased, the strengths often go from poor to good rather quickly, especially in the case of wildland firefighters because they enter training beat up and detrained after a long fire season. It is much easier for an athlete to reacquire skills and physical capacities compared to the time and effort it takes to learn and develop new skills and capacities. Sierra was no different in this regard even though she was a city firefighter. She was out of shape, at least according to her own standards. She did have what sounded like substantial endurance capabilities at one time. I hoped that we could reignite her!

Detraining occurs when an athlete stops training or decreases training volume, intensity, or both. For wildland firefighters, this often occurs during fire season, and by the end of the season, they are in a detrained state. Physically, they are incapable of performing at the level of capacity they entered the season.

I had two realizations about Sierra—one, that she was talented, and two, that she was going to be difficult to train. Her wine and dine lifestyle would hopefully change for the better as the difficulty and volume of training increased. She lacked requisite upper body strength, and over the years of her firefighting career, she had learned that she was physically talented and capable of scraping by on her ability alone. She didn't have to train with a detailed, periodized, and consistent weekly fitness regimen or eat particularly well. I had seen this with naturally talented athletes in the past. They seem to work hard at what they are good at, and they get by on that main skill or ability, but they also have difficulty improving upon their weaker aspects because their strengths came so easily that they never had to feel the pain of the learning process. I had succeeded as an athlete for many years relying on this strategy. I knew it well.

This attitude would have to change for her to be successful. I couldn't see how anyone, especially a female approaching forty, could show up and scrape by. She would have to embrace the learning process, the feeling of sucking at something and being ok with showing up each day while continuing to suck for a long while.

Also stacked against her was a case of hip bursitis, which Sierra mentioned before we began the first week of training. Hip bursitis is best treated with rest and physical therapy, and if still persistent, then with a corticosteroid injection (cortisone, for example). We couldn't afford to sacrifice training time to rest and wait for this to heal, so I decided to proceed cautiously with her running volume, and I planned to write in extra hip mobility and stability training to combat the issue. Hopefully that would be enough. If this got worse over the training season, it could jeopardize everything.

Her natural endurance ability was something special, though. In her life, she had run some ultramarathons and was not worried in the slightest about the long distances the rookie trainers may demand of her. She was concerned about her running speed for the 1.5-mile test, her strength for the calisthenic tests and subsequent volume blasting with pull-ups, push-ups, sit-ups, and other core-taxing tasks, and of course, the heavy hikes. That 110-pound pack was very heavy for her, and she was concerned about it. And rightly so. These were her weaknesses, and we had a short time to change them from liabilities into assets.

With most females, physical size is a factor due to the strength requirements of rookie training. At 5'6" and 135 lbs., Sierra is larger than Heidi, but she is still significantly smaller than the male rookies that she'd be competing against for a position as a smokejumper, especially if she lost another 10 pounds.

After a few more conversations and further tinkering to decipher her current physical abilities and how to best structure her training to fit her numerous schedule and time demands, we began the six-month trek towards rookie training.

PLANNING HER PROGRAM

A few days after first speaking with Sierra, I sat at my kitchen table and prepared to write the initial days of her training program. I like to begin the season planning process by working backwards, as I did with Heidi, like Mike and I did with the Illinois track and field athletes. I figure out where I want my athlete or team to physically and mentally be at the end of their season and then work backwards logically and linearly from there until I arrive at today. It's always a best guess, and the more athletes and teams you work with, the better your estimation becomes, to an extent. Considering the complexity of Sierra's living situation and nonlinear full-time job, I saw no possible way to create a detailed plan for the next 6 months. Instead, I planned to rely on programming out in short spurts. I was not good at this, yet.

Even though training would be nonlinear and unpredictable, I hoped that significantly improving Sierra's physical skills was still possible. I would have to be on my game with monitoring weekly and monthly progress to ensure that we stuck roughly to the potential trajectories for each task. I would not be able to plan out her program a month in advance. Planning would have to be a weekly endeavor, and sometimes daily. To enhance the effectiveness of this unique approach, we would have to adopt clear and honest communication. I vowed to work each week to get to know her better as a person and an athlete. I asked her to communicate clearly and openly with me. Armed with my computer and notebook and surrounded by the chaos of boxes and clothing strewn about, I drafted a simple approach.

With Heidi, I had trained her firsthand for a few months years before we worked together in preparation for Boise, so I had some idea of what she was capable of. With Sierra, I had no idea how she moved. I had never worked with her. She had little experience with barbell training. Her kettlebell experience was also minimal, and I was uncertain of the movement quality of her basic bodyweight tasks like squatting and hinging. This is risky. Asking an athlete to perform increasingly high repetition volumes can cause overuse injuries if not performed with sound technique. In addition, I had worked with some athletes in the past who were endurance specialists, and they moved very poorly outside the sport of running. I hoped that Sierra would move better than them. She would have to!

ROOKIE TRAINING STANDARDS

Even though Sierra was not yet accepted as a smokejumper candidate, we used the Redding standards as initial targets. Redding is a US Forest Service base, so there are no "high standards." That didn't stop Sierra from setting lofty goals. After thinking back to Heidi's experience through three different rookie trainings, I thought that lofty goals were exactly the right approach. Heidi had emphasized being able to hit the minimum PT standards was simply "a snowflake on the tip of the iceberg," meaning that candidates should aim high to blow the minimum standards out of the water while preparing for the most challenging experience of their lives. While Sierra was currently close to the minimum standards, I believed that she had much room for improvement.

To begin the detailed planning process, I suggested that Sierra perform a full PT test minus the 110-pound pack carry and send me the data. It's always a good to see exactly where the athletes are at the start instead of blindly estimating their abilities. Here were her marks:

	USFS Standards	*Sierra's Initial Goals*	*Sierra's preseason scores*
1.5-mile Run	11:00	9:00	10:00
Pull-ups	7	15	6
Push-ups	45	75	48
Sit-ups	100	100	86
Pack Test	110 lbs., 3 miles, 90 minutes	60:00:00	no result, yet

For the 1.5-mile run, she was about one minute faster than the Redding standard, and one minute slower than her goal of 9:00. I was not concerned about her running ability in the slightest. However, I was concerned about her strength. Even though she was physically larger than Heidi, her strength was far behind. On the pull-ups, she was one rep shy of the minimum standard and three push-ups beyond the standard. Her sit-ups were also below the minimum standard, and she had no best mark on the 110-pound ruck.

We had quite a bit of work to do, but I was confident that Sierra had the right combination of physical ability to make it through rookie training. I was not yet familiar with her mindset, though, and as I learned with Heidi, mindset in this realm is everything. You can have the fittest athletes on the planet fail a physical challenge if they have chinks in their mindset. Sierra was about to get hers tested.

I assumed that Sierra was mentally strong. One does not run 50+ miles with a weak mind or body. However, rookie training would be a different beast. There would be some running, but it's not a running race. She'd be in boots and often carrying a pack and a QB (a large plastic cube filled with water), and sometimes a saw or Pulaski. There would be tree climbing and thousands of reps of pull-ups, push-ups, sit-ups, and other core-fatiguing varieties like what Heidi experienced at Boise. There would be mid-hike lunges, squats, and burpees, and cutting line for hours on end.

I'd had a taste of success with Heidi, and I wanted Sierra to be successful, too. Even though this was her first attempt at smokejumper rookie training, might as well get it right the first time. Heidi had had some serious mental barriers to overcome from her previous experiences at rookie training. It was a benefit for Sierra to go into the selection process without knowing how hard it was going to be. To learn more about Sierra's mindset, I began to dig. I sought to better understand the woman that I was committed to working with for the next six months.

When assessing how to train an athlete, it's helpful to get an idea of who the person is that you're training. What are their goals? How good do they think they are compared to reality? How do they move? How do they stack up to other athletes in their field? How cerebral are they? What are their strengths and weaknesses? Taking that a step further, when coaching an athlete to accomplish something massive, you must shift from coaching the physical to the mental and psychological. You must learn as much as possible about their mindset by asking the right questions and listening to their answers, and from those answers finding further questions to ask and buttons to push to dig even deeper. You must have the courage to ask the questions, knowing full well that you will receive pushback. You might even have to fight. If you don't dig, you may leave some stones unturned and unrealized gains on the table. You must learn what makes them tick.

I learned how to dig into the minds of athletes in college when observing my track coaches and how they worked to influence my teammates during high pressure track meets, and how they communicated with me during decathlons, which are intense and heavily physically, mentally, and emotionally draining experiences. My first season, I noticed that they rarely dug deep enough to get below my emotional smokescreen, and I paid the price by falling short of expectations. In the next few years, they dug deeper, and I eventually let them in. Together, we worked through my mindset issues, and the result was two consecutive national championships.

When an athlete has a massive goal and has asked you to coach them, you must get into their head, and they must voluntarily choose to become vulnerable enough to let you in. With an athlete like Sierra, if you don't thoroughly scour their psychology to uncover where they are weak, compassionately reflect this to back to them, and then help them address their weaknesses, the sheer volume and intensity of rookie training and the rookie trainers who run the process will expose those weaknesses through physical fatigue, and they will crush her.

Crushed doesn't necessarily mean just psychologically upset her so that she washes out. The danger of smokejumper rookie training should not be underestimated. It is not uncommon for less than half to make it through rookie training each year. Sometimes, candidates are hospitalized. I have even heard of washed rookies who are still physically broken and recovering from the experience a year or more afterwards. This fact alone clearly illustrates the severity.

After my initial phone call with Sierra and some subsequent calls to iron out the details for training, I sat down at my kitchen table on a Saturday in late October 2017 and drafted an initial training program. I created a spreadsheet for us to utilize, and on it, I devised a more streamlined approach to breaking up her training tabs. The first tab to the bottom left was titled "General Planning," and that's where I placed my psychological assessment. I put some get-to-know-you questions there and made a place for her to respond:

Sierra's Psychological Self-assessment: "I tend to lack focus and I tend to have too much going on in my life."

My coaching approach: Give Sierra a task list that can be done in any order, any day, any time. Fritz programs. Sierra works when she sees fit.

Sierra's Psychological Self-assessment: "I also struggle with my eating and drinking habits. I drink beer or wine in the evening or with dinner every night that I'm not working. I tend to eat big dinners and nothing during the day. I've always been this way."

My coaching approach: "This may not be a problem, yet. However, your weight loss will occur more rapidly if you reduce or cut out the alcohol. You may need to replace it with a healthy habit instead."

Sierra's Psychological Self-assessment: "I used to drink and smoke and party pretty hard and then show up for work and hike the saw up the hill faster than everyone. I did that for years. I can be a little extreme. I have a hard time with order and schedules. Sometimes I think I lack dedication but at the same time I have a lot of accomplishments. I have 2 undergrad degrees and a masters and I'm working on a second masters now. I also managed to pass the academy for San Diego which was incredibly challenging. I don't know how I've scraped by!"

My coaching approach: "Haha, I feel similar to you. I have a bachelors' and two master's degrees, but I still am figuring out my life and what I'm going to do for the rest of it! Just from talking with you, I assume that you have "scraped by" because you like to be a badass. You work harder than others. You're impulsive, which is a double-edged sword. One side allows you to act without hesitation. The other side is a lack of consistency and diligence, perhaps."

Sierra seemed honest, hardworking, humble, and chaotic. She liked variety, and she enjoyed long bouts of endurance feats. She stayed very busy, and it seemed to me that she enjoyed the lack of predicable, repetitive structure. Her training would have to mirror this. Due to her success in ultra-endurance events across the spectrum of human movement, I gathered that she was extremely competitive.

Here is a list of Sierra's best running performance data which she sent to me for reference. The list includes some event results:

- Ran 2 miles in 12 minutes on a treadmill. This is 6:00/mile pace, which is fast enough for her to run about 9:00 in the 1-5-mile for the PT test. I was unsure of how recently she was able to run at this pace.
- For the San Diego Fire Academy, Sierra ran a 19-minute 5k, which comes out to 6:07/mile pace.
- A 41-minute 10k, which comes out to 6:36/mile. This is plenty fast enough for a smokejumper. With this pace, she'd be near the front of most packs. For reference, Army Rangers must run 5 miles in 35 minutes or less, which is 7:00/mile pace.
- She had run a few 50-mile races:
    - In the summer of 2016, she won first for the females in The Pioneer Spirit, a 50-mile race, taking 6th overall.
    - In the Kodiak 50-miler, she took 3rd place.
    - In the Avalon 50-miler on Catalina Island, she took 4th place

She also had a few other impressive accomplishments:

- She had competed in and placed with the top finishers for ocean swims and duathlons. A duathlon is like a triathlon, but instead of swimming, there is another running leg (run-bike-run)

- She once completed a 12-mile non-stop open ocean swim.
- She held the world record for the largest spearfish-caught Calico Bass.

I unpacked all of that and combined it with what I already knew about her. She had (at least in the past, she said she as overweight) the ability at one point to run at a 6:00 mile pace for 2 miles, a 6:07 pace for three miles, and a 6:36 pace for just over 6 miles straight. She could also run fast enough over 50-mile distances to win or place highly in those races. She was a strong swimmer and had incredible lungs. Once, I asked her how deep she spearfished, and she said about 20 meters. That's 66 feet under water in the ocean. And she wasn't even using an oxygen tank. That's on a breath hold. I asked her how long she could hold her breath. She responded, "while spearfishing, for over three minutes." That is remarkable. Holding one's breath while not moving for three minutes is very challenging. A three-minute breath hold while hunting fish at the bottom of the ocean with a spear gun is something else entirely.

Her pull-ups needed a lot of work. She was currently at 6 strict pull-ups with a goal of 15 reps by the start of rookie training, which was now less than six months away. Going from 6 reps to 15 would be a crazy feat in that amount of time. Her push-up goal was also lofty, moving from her current best mark of 48 reps to 75. I hoped that we had enough time for her to improve these marks. Even if she achieved those massive PT personal bests, she would be entering rookie training with considerably less strength endurance than Heidi. Sierra did have an ace in the hole—her immense endurance capacity. That gift is something you can't teach.

I instinctually felt that Sierra's endurance ability would go the distance. Even now, before undergoing the long trek towards rookie training, she probably had plenty to make it through. However, I was concerned that she would succumb to the heavy carries and thousands of calisthenics. She simply did not yet have the volume exposure and tolerance to those tasks. She needed to get stronger. A lot stronger. And she needed to build her muscle endurance specific to the physical tasks that she might encounter.

Next, I put on my programming hat. As I sat piecing everything together, I realized that I didn't have to improve Sierra's endurance capacity, which was a relief. She could already run very long distances, and her body could recover from immense volume training, meaning that she could tolerate high volume running work. I had a feeling that we could translate this to hiking ability rather easily by getting her stronger.

As I pondered how to train Sierra, I thought back to my old coach and roommate, Mike. He and I would often discuss hypothetical athletes, training possibilities, probabilities, and the limits of human performance. Natural ability was one of our frequent conversations. In long distance running, to win at the division I level and beyond, often the top athletes are putting in 100-120 miles of distance A WEEK, and sometimes longer. The theory is that running volume provides adaptations to running efficiency and physiology which produce national and world champions. Athletes who run less distance than this simply cannot push their VO2 max high enough to compete with the humans who are able to handle those insane training volumes.

This example illustrates the sheer volume requirements of the human body to produce the fastest endurance athletes. Mike and I hypothesized that if you took 10,000 (or even 100,000, or a million) people and had them all run a hundred miles in a week, 99.99% of them would break in some way. An overuse injury of some type would result. However, that 00.01% of those 10,000 people would handle that training volume due to genetic factors. Perhaps their joints are structured in a way to bear load symmetrically and efficiently through immense mechanical stress. Their muscles might have the right fiber type distribution to support the demands of running 100+ miles in a week. In general, they just had the ability to do a shit-ton of repetitive physical work without breaking. This is arguably an innate talent, a genetic gift, like people who can naturally jump high, sprint ridiculously fast, or lift extremely heavy things.

I believed that Sierra was in this 00.01% of natural ability to handle a high workload without breaking down. Combined with an active lifetime and coming from a family of ultra-endurance athletes, she had been training for this her entire life. Over the next six months, we were about to put this hypothesis to the test.

Muscle fiber distribution. Muscle fibers can be categorized as Type I or Type II. Type I fibers are "slow twitch," meaning they fire slowly and are fatigue resistant and are great for endurance tasks. Type II "fast twitch" muscle fibers are larger in diameter and produce a faster rate of firing. They fatigue more quickly than Type I fibers, but before they do, they produce a lot more force. They are the muscle fibers that support fast, explosive, and heavy tasks like weightlifting, carrying heavy things, sprinting, jumping, throwing, punching, kicking. The fun stuff.

END OF OCTOBER 2017

I started Sierra on her training during the last week of October in 2017. As with Heidi, I sent all the training to Sierra, and she completed the work on her own, a completely remote coach-athlete relationship. I had not met her in person, yet. Over the first few weeks of training, I found it difficult to get in step with her, perhaps because she lived so much faster than I was living, even though I felt like I was living a mile a minute. Everything was in flux for me. Jess and I had just moved down to San Diego. We'd found a rental house. It was small, painted blue, and sat at the back of a property that had three other little casitas in a row to the left. The yard was full of grass and trees, and our house had an accompanying garage. The unit was a great price, and the landlord made snarky jokes about everything during that first encounter. He toured us through the place, boasting, "Welcome to this spacious 750-square-foot three-bedroom house in a quiet and up-and-coming neighborhood..." It wasn't quiet or up-and-coming. It wasn't spacious. And it had one real bedroom. The second "bedroom" was a 6 x 6' closet with a window taking up the entire wall, and the third room was an 8 x 9' Tetris-piece-shaped mud room with a door to the alleyway at the back of the house that must have been a porch once and had since been poorly enclosed. Neither of those rooms could house guests or roommates. They were too small or awkwardly shaped to fit a bed larger than a shoebox. Later, we found out from our first neighbor that the entire development had been erected almost ninety years before and used as a dormitory for people who built the San Diego World Fair in 1935.

I thought the landlord was a riot. Jess didn't find him as funny. She loves stand-up comedy, so I guess the guy's jokes weren't hitting hard enough. We almost found a new place after seeing him kick at and chase a large white cat out of the yard and grumbled about calling animal control. That pesky cat was always lurking around, he said.

Even though the neighborhood wasn't great, we decided it was a decent fit for our first location in San Diego. Plus, we really didn't know which neighborhoods were good, yet. The real draw of the place was the front porch. It was tucked behind a small pear tree and a blossoming Bougainvillea bush. I planned to spend much of my time on that lovely porch.

While Jess brought home the bacon working at the hospital, I worked diligently to maintain coaching relationships with some of my athletes from Redlands. I wrote them training each week and used video coaching to critique their form. This brought in a little bit of money. With no physical job lined up in San Diego, I had no place to go during the day. In Redlands, I had been working long days with very little time off, so this experience felt freeing. I needed the rest. I was the main financial provider in Redlands for years. This was my first break in a long while. I was sure it would grow old fast though.

When Jess was off from work, we explored San Diego. Everything was 10–15 minutes from our place. Beaches, bars, restaurants, hiking. We'd walk the entire length of Coronado beach, and afterwards, grab a beer at a local brewery. When we lived in Redlands, every week, we had a Friday lunch date at a place called Eureka Burger. That's where Jess and I learned about beer. Sure, we had each drunk thousands in college, but those were Coors Light. At Eureka, we'd gotten to know the bartender, who'd slowly exposed our taste buds to the large and expanding world of craft beer. Reds, browns, Belgians, IPA's, and eventually sours. Jessica hated IPAs at first. By the end of our last year in Redlands, she'd become a kind of a snob about them. Our bartender was also a pastor. And an actor. And rode a motorcycle. Quite the mixture of things. We asked him to be our officiant at our wedding before we left. He gladly accepted.

Jess's schedule in San Diego was unpredictable, and she ended up working a lot of weekends. On those weekends, I often took the 90-minute drive up to Redlands to train a handful of athletes at a colleague's gym to make a few hundred dollars. I would stay with friends in Redlands on Saturday night, drinking wine, eating cheese, talking about life, and planning the future. On Sunday, I'd drive back home and post up in the back mudroom which I'd converted into my office. That's where I did my programming. No more oversized kitchen table. Instead, I purchased a faux mahogany desk from Target, the kind a college kid would use to write essays. That's where I would program from now on.

Sierra's first week of training was upon us. For the first few days, I started her out with low volume bodyweight and lightly loaded training, and I did my best to tailor her tasks each day to where she physically was—the firehouse, one of the boats, or up in Forest Falls. She completed her strength work mostly at the fire station. Sierra would tell me what her next week of work and life looked like, and I did my best to adapt the training to her. She loved to get in the ocean, so on her off days, I structured some free time in the ocean which she enjoyed. She swam or surfed. She completed yoga for recovery.

On day three, Saturday, October 28, she was scheduled to go lobster diving and spear fishing, but instead at the last minute, she called an audible and had to finish up some things for her master's program. I guess she felt the need to celebrate and went out and partied that night for Halloween. The next day, she completed a six-hour trail run. In the spreadsheets, she wrote, "Amazing run today. I felt great even after a halloween drunk fest last night! I ran from my house up to the summit of San G. I had to walk a 2 mile section at the top but may have had a PR for my San G time (although I've never timed it before)." She continued, "I didn't stop once not even for water or to eat at the top. it was 24 miles and took me 5 hours 58 minutes. Its a very difficult run and makes me think i'm ready to be placing in a 50 soon! Even with my fat bod I got up there pretty quick and my hip and calf didn't hurt at all. Amazing! My legs do feel tired though, but my fatigue was minimal."

I unpacked that feedback paragraph. I knew about her hip, but her comment that there was no calf pain immediately placed that issue on my coaching radar. Any joint or tissue that is sensitive to an athlete, the coach must be hyper-aware when programming training tasks. Secondly, she ran for 6 hours with no food and only a little water. That itself is extreme, impressive, and of course, dangerous. The "hike" that she went on is one of the toughest in the area. San G is short for San Gorgonio. The locals call it Old Greyback. The peak is 11,500 feet, the tallest in Southern California. From Forest Falls via the Vivian Creek Trail, the hike is 19 miles out and back and covers almost 5,500 feet of elevation gain (that's more than a mile of vert). She must have started the hike from her cabin, adding a few miles to each leg of the hike. I completed this hike with friends a few years ago, and it was a very tough hike for me, and I was strong at the time. I guess my endurance was not up to Sierra's level.

Go figure. I couldn't believe that she ran most of the way up and down. On my way up, for the last mile, I walked slow as an old man, and it felt like I was breathing through a straw. On the way back down, my knees were so swollen that I had to use hiking poles during the last thousand-foot descent into Forest Falls as we ran out of daylight.

The next day after her trek up San G, I designated her to rest, thinking that she would need some time off to recover. She did rest, but in her own way. She spent five hours that day "bucking with a chainsaw" (bucking is cutting up felled trees into shorter lengths) and split so much wood with an axe that afterwards, her cabin was prepared with firewood for the entire winter! In the same week, she began complaining that I was having her rest too much and that she was used to training daily. I told her that rest was a weapon when used properly and that we'd pick up training soon. It was only the first few days of week one, after all.

Within that first week, I also had Sierra take the 3-mile flat pack test with 45 pounds to get an initial time. She completed this in just under 34 minutes, which is about 11-minute mile pace. This was blazing fast, so I had a feeling that we could increase weight more rapidly than I had with Heidi. Plus, Sierra's body was not as run down as Heidi's had been. Sierra was also physically larger, so 45 pounds for her was not as heavy as 45 pounds was for Heidi. In addition, Sierra wasn't coming off a tough wildland fire season. Her current structural firefighting job was demanding in a much different way compared to wildland fire. If we upped the pack weight quickly, I knew that Sierra's lungs could handle it. However, I was concerned about where and how her strength would begin to limit her progress and if her hip or calf would act up.

On Saturday, November 4, I had written Sierra a recovery day. Swim for 30 minutes and take an hour-long easy bike ride. Simple enough. Instead, she swam 2700 meters (over an hour of swimming) and ran 10 miles (about an hour and a half of running). This was the first true instance that I knew she was going to be challenging to coach. When I read her feedback, I threw my hands in the air with a grunt and leaned back in my chair. How was I supposed to plan any progressions for her if she did whatever she felt like on any given day? I complained to Jess, and she laughed and shook her head, and said, "She's gonna get hurt. Tell her to stick to the plan!" Ahh, Jess with her matter-of-fact problem-solving skills. She especially loved playing armchair quarterback to solve my professional and personal problems. It infuriated me every time.

It would be reasonable for an athlete to swim an extra 10 minutes or bike a little further than planned and say that they felt good and didn't want to stop. Sierra, on the other hand, would add extra hours to her training or go on a long run and skip an entire day of training. This was incredibly frustrating to me. We were only two weeks in, and already, I was pulling my hair out. If I had longer or tougher training planned for the next day, now I had to go into the spreadsheets and push that back a few days or delete it completely.

For one, this was a ton of extra work, and two, I was concerned about her getting injured. To top it all off, I did a poor job of communicating my frustrations to Sierra. I felt like I didn't yet know her well enough to be hard on her. Part of me wanted to demand that she follow training exactly as I wrote it, but there was a small voice in my head that questioned whether that would work with her. It might push her away. I also took into consideration that she had successfully run ultramarathons and placed at the top, and her body had held together through those events and the training leading up to them. That suggested she knew how to listen to her body. I was torn. When in doubt, sometimes it's best to make minimal adjustments. So that's what I did. I kept asking her to stick to the plan and hoped that she would. I didn't go over the top and lose my shit, even though I wanted to. Sierra was a wild mustang and I had not yet tamed her. Perhaps she was not meant to be tamed. I didn't want her to run completely wild, though. Left to her own devices, I thought she would choose distance running only and might not hit enough PT volume to prepare for rookie training.

NOVEMBER 2017

I was now settling into San Diego. Jess worked a shift that started at 5 p.m. She woke at noon to start her day. We'd sit on the front porch hidden from the street by the small pear tree and the Bougainvillea bush to pass the time before she headed to the hospital. Jess drank her coffee and I'd sit in the sun. I didn't drink coffee. It made me too hyper. One of Jess's favorite jabs against me when I am caffeinated is, "too many words, not enough thoughts." So, I sat silently and enjoyed the weather, which was still warm this time of year. While sitting on the porch, that large white cat came up and rubbed itself on my leg, purring. I was hesitant at first to pet him because he looked rough. Like a street cat that had been in all the fights. This was the same cat that the landlord had chased away. According to our neighbor, people called the cat Jumbo or Dumb-Dumb. He was a stray and looked like a ghost, with his face all swollen from who knows what. Fights, parasites, a hard life on the street. The poor thing looked sickly. Apparently, the cat's owner used to live in one of the other casitas on the property and had moved out a year ago, abandoning this poor cat and his younger sister to fend for themselves. The sister didn't make it, and Jumbo was all alone. He seemed sweet enough. He was like a dog. If you whistled or clicked your tongue at him, he would jog over and nuzzle into you. If you sat back and tapped your thighs, he'd hop right up on your lap. Smart boy. After a few weeks of getting to know him, we realized that he was a big sweetheart. Despite his weathered appearance, Jess and I immediately fell for him.

Here we were five years after moving from Illinois to Redlands, and we had changed everything in our lives once more. To top it all off, we were in the wedding planning process, which was now six months away. Jessica was enjoying her job, for the most part. She was learning the ropes at her busy hospital. She said it was much busier than anywhere she had trained during her degree program. She was welcomed in by the older crew of women who made up most of her colleagues. She only came home in tears occasionally. The first month was very challenging for her, and I wouldn't even be awake to console her. She really didn't need consoling, though. Even if I woke up and tried to hold her or ask questions, she would want her space. "I'm fine," she'd say and she'd shut down. Perhaps this was the toughest lesson that I learned about her, that she didn't need me around. Sure, I'd hear what happened the next day on our walk, but she was as disinterested in my opinion on how she could have handled her own work situation as I was on hearing how she'd coach Sierra.

Sierra wanted to do it all. She felt like competing in a 50-mile ultra-endurance event this off-season, but I suggested that this didn't fit with her needs for her preparation. We knew that she had incredible endurance ability, but she lacked strength. This is where we needed to spend the most time working. I did my best to convey the body's limited recovery capacity. Every human has a finite amount of physical work that they can complete and recover from. If we trained for long running, there would be less "recovery dollars" left over to repair damage from strength training, where it's needed most. In other words, her strength training improvements would trickle in slowly. In addition, running too fast or too far on a Tuesday would decrease her ability to perform quality strength training the next day, and sometimes a day after that. This was a hard lesson that she and I both unfortunately learned multiple times over the course of our coaching relationship.

One of the toughest things that a coach must do is save an athlete from themselves. As athletes, when left to our own devices, we often self limit due to our own biases and an inability to take a step back and look at ourselves more objectively. That was my job as Sierra's coach—to help round out her training. I was doing my best, but it felt like I was failing.

Our plan to play her programming by ear each day was holding up like a plane taped together with duct tape. Sierra sometimes switched training days around, which wasn't too much of an issue, yet. However, she continued to do much more work than I intended her to do. This was becoming problematic. She wasn't fighting me. It wasn't malicious. It simply felt like she got into the flow of certain tasks, mainly long runs and swims, and would take them for miles or hours longer than seemed beneficial from my more objective vantage point as coach.

Sierra wrote, "Today I ran 10 miles before I did this workout. I was feeling good so I ran." I smiled and shook my head. This was the first instance when she went way beyond what I had written. I suggested that she complete a 20-minute dynamic warm-up and even spelled out which tasks to complete, and instead, she ran 10 miles which probably took her over an hour and a half.

I patiently worked towards educating her on how I plan and program, and when appropriate, showed how her extra work negatively affected the next day of training. I constantly debated how to communicate with her about how each change that she made affected future training and the overall trajectory of her progress.

I knew that she wasn't adding more work to her training sessions out of some ego-driven desire to prove to me that she could handle more work. I knew that she could handle more work. However, I also knew that more was not the answer. Many athletes assume that more is better. Oftentimes, it's not. Better was the answer.

I learned that more is not better by injuring myself constantly as a young athlete. After relearning this lesson multiple times across different injuries in various areas of my body, eventually I realized that more is not better. Better is better. And as a coach or an athlete, once you can identify what better looks like, then you can begin to program towards that. Furthermore, athletes, when left to their own devices, will often do what they like and not necessarily what they need. They are enshrouded in the trees and cannot see the forest. Once again, that is my job—to see the forest, paint it, and then zoom in layering individual brush strokes to each tree, mushroom, rock, and plant.

In my opinion, Sierra needed to distribute her training time and recovery resources towards improving her weaker areas, namely strength endurance specific to the PT test and all the other various PT tasks that she would be exposed to in rookie training.

Progress was occurring despite sparse communication. During the first week of November, she completed the heavy pack training at 55 pounds, 10 pounds heavier than the week before, in just under 36 minutes. She was still improving rapidly with this task, which was a relief. At work, she would play ultimate frisbee and tracked her distance during matches at around 3 miles, some of which was sprinting and change of direction. I made sure to factor this work into her training volume each week. I hoped that the ultimate frisbee would help with her 1.5-mile speed. It wasn't directly 1.5-mile preparation, but it was better than nothing.

Still without a smokejumper candidate offer, Sierra was now looking at jumping out of Fairbanks, Alaska. That was a BLM base, and the standards were higher than at Redding. This didn't stop her from wanting it all. After a short sprint day to help increase her running speed, I wrote in a rest day followed by a long trail run. She wrote, "Only ran 21 miles. My legs had a lot of lactic acid buildup from either the sprints or weight vest bear crawls. I had to walk a lot of the uphill sections and then it was getting dark so I had to stop. It was a beautiful run and i spend a lot of time visualizing during Long runs. I ran the first section of the PCT from the border to lake morena ... I think I will still finish the 50 fine but maybe not be winning it as I had hoped!"

I had mixed feelings about her training performance. I was happy to receive so much feedback from her. I wasn't happy to hear that she had to cut her long run short due to feeling the effects of our strength training. This told me that she was prioritizing her long runs over calisthenics. Of course, she would accumulate more soreness from our strength training sessions compared to her running. Strength was newer to her, and she had a deficit that we were working to overcome. However, I was thrilled to hear that she was experimenting with visualization on her own! She didn't share what she visualized on her long run. I was curious, though. Throughout the first month, I had written her a few mental training prompts in the spreadsheets at the top of each training day, and each week they remained blank. At least she was exploring some mindset training on her own.

To improve her absolute strength to help keep her improving on the heavy pack work, I wrote in barbell deadlifts on weeks that she had access to the barbells at work or at her Forest Falls cabin. And since we both now lived in San Diego, we agreed to meet up so I could check her technique. I had outfitted my old, tiny, rickety, termite-riddled, boarded-up garage with a piece of turf and some equipment and figured that training Sierra was a good way to break in the space. Even though we had been working together for over a month now, I felt the flutters in my stomach a few minutes before she arrived to train.

This was my first experience meeting a client in person whom I had only interacted with through phone calls, texts, and dialogue in the training spreadsheets. When she arrived, we shared an awkward greeting, unsure how to interact. Perhaps she expected me to be different, and maybe I thought that she would be as well. It's difficult to gage personality and chemistry over the phone and through a spreadsheet. Upon first meeting me, I can seem stoic and lack enthusiasm. Sierra seemed a bit distant, like she was still deciding how much to trust me.

My assessment started with a general warm-up, and I watched her move through it. While I sized her up, I felt like I was also being evaluated. I gave her the same warm-up tasks that she should have been completing on her own. When she didn't know what some of them were, I asked her what she was doing instead to warm up. Breaking the tension, Sierra laughed and said that she usually doesn't, or she runs. Relaxing a bit, I laughed as well, knowing full well she wasn't warming up. I suggested that she warm up from now on, and when any questions arose about the tasks I wrote, to text me and I could send her a demo video or explain the value of the drill.

From the assessment, I gathered that Sierra moved well enough. When athletes can squat or hinge, the next worthwhile conversation is tension. They might look like they are moving well, but are they engaging the right muscles at the right time to keep them safe and enable a progression of strength, and how conscious of these connections are they? How are they breathing, and where is their balance? Sierra and I spent the latter half of that first session working to create proper tension to support breathing and bracing while swinging a kettlebell, and eventually, squatting. I also tested her push-ups and pull-up technique to make sure the rookie trainers would accept her range of motion. They looked good.

Even though Sierra had been running fast and far for years, she had a young training age for "gym" tasks. She moved well despite a lack of understanding in creating appropriate tension, and by the end of the session, Sierra had loosened up and began to laugh more freely at my coaching explanations and quips as she began to consider my coaching and allowed herself to make some mistakes that I was able to correct. This was one small step in the right direction for improving our coach/athlete relationship.

Ten days before the end of this second training month, Sierra completed a 65-pound pack test, a 10-pound jump from the previous heavy pack training. This was the heaviest pack yet. I was progressing her quickly to see what she could handle. She was still feeling her hip bursitis, but it seemed to be improving. However, I still didn't think that she was completely warming up or cooling down from her training because later that day when hitting her strength training, her knee began to act up.

While this could be due to old age (she was pushing towards 40, after all, and currently training like a mid-twenties professional athlete), I had not heard Sierra complain about her knees before. It made me wonder whether she was being as thorough as she could with her pre- and post-training body upkeep. I saw this feedback about knee discomfort and remembered that Sierra was developing a habit of not warming up beforehand and not cooling down after training sessions. Or at least that's how it seemed from scanning the spreadsheet and from our first in-person coaching session. The feedback cells in the warm-up and cooldown sections of her training were still empty. Everywhere. Sometimes the importance of specific tasks like a diligent adherence to warm-up and cooldown habits may slip through the cracks. With Sierra, perhaps I didn't stress the importance of a full warm-up and cooldown each day. I think that it was easier for Heidi to commit herself to these habits because she was a full-time athlete, and I tied the healing of Heidi's plantar fasciitis to consistency in these actions. For Sierra, she was busy with her full-time job and master's program. However, I felt that wasn't a good excuse because of what Sierra had on the line. If she went into rookie training physically banged up, she wouldn't last a single day.

In our shared training spreadsheets, I provide detailed warm-ups for each day, and I created five different warm-up variations to keep the process interesting and novel. It had worked for Heidi, so I assumed that it would also work for Sierra. Years before, as a coach in the track and field world, I saw that Tonja prepared different warm-ups for each day and that giving athletes the same warm-up day after day becomes monotonous to them, which defeats one of the main purposes of the warm-up, which is to align the athlete's mind with their body for the session ahead. Performing the same warm-up day in and day out can cause athletes to "go through the motions." I noticed that over the past month of training together, Sierra had stopped writing her feedback next to each warm-up section. It felt like she was going through the motions.

Lucky for us both, the day after her knee acted up, it felt fine again, and she was able to hit full training with no restrictions. Great timing, too, because her ultra-endurance race was coming up in a week and a half. Sierra was headed to Arizona for a 50-mile race at the beginning of December. I didn't want to peak her for this race by heavily cutting down training volume because that would significantly slow her progress towards rookie training. I also didn't want her going into this ultramarathon too busted up because that could be dangerous, so we couldn't keep pushing her PT training full speed. I decided to decrease her training volume a little bit and added in some strategic rest two days before her race. I created a simple shakeout training session the day before her event so she could work out the aches and pains that had settled in during her long drive to the event.

I wasn't completely comfortable with Sierra competing in this race because it slowed the progress of our training and unnecessarily risked her physical health, but I also understood that she loved running these races and we still had a little over four months to prepare. That is, if she received a candidate bid. She was still training on faith that she would get an offer to smokejump next year.

DECEMBER 2017

Jess's favorite month was here, December. No, it wasn't her birthday month. That's in March. And she does treat the entire month as her birthday, constantly reminding me that it's her birthday month and that she can do whatever she wants. No, the month of December is Christmas month. Jess loves Christmas. On December 6, apparently Santa Claus was born, and Jess reminds me of this every year by playing the song which celebrates this marvelous day while she dances around in her pajamas after waking up at noon.

December is a tough month for me because it adds hours to my schedule and dozens of items to my "honey-do" list. I had two full days of programming to complete each week, and now I had to hang Christmas lights and lug trees around and whatnot, all at the beck and call of my wife to be. Deep down, I loved it. But I would never tell her that. I'd trounce around complaining and swearing away, breaking things around the house, sometimes on purpose. I think she secretly knows I love how much she loves Christmas even though she fervently calls me a grinch every single year.

Despite some ups through this magical month, I felt unmotivated to program, exercise, shop, cook, or clean. Jess was still the main breadwinner, so it was my job to keep the home in order. I had become a house husband. For Christmas that year, Jess even gifted me a pretty cooking apron. Perhaps that was her way of saying, "go get a job and make some real money." I was getting fat, too. San Diego was tough on me. Leaving Redlands was still a sore spot. I missed being a man of the town. In San Diego, I felt like a twig in a rainforest.

My San Diego blues didn't bode well for optimally supporting Sierra. Even though there is a science to programming, it feels more like art. It's creative, a blending of math, movement, and strategic planning. And to create art, one needs to be present. I knew this because a lifetime ago (in college, about 12 years ago), I has been a studio art major, burning the candle at both ends every day, for years, and loving every minute of it. I was a potter, and I sculpted and painted. I know how my creativity sparks, and it's not when I was feeling like this. Even my athlete's feedback on weeks when I feel down seem like the world is coming to an end. At least we had that damned white cat living in the yard.

Hanging out on the porch with that flea-ridden bumfighter was the highlight of my evenings at home when Jess was at work. One chilly and sunny December day, Jess and I sat out on the front porch. We had purchased a small rickety table and chairs, and the white cat was spread out across the top of the entire table, soaking up the sun. While petting him, Jess and I saw a worm crawling around on his little cat butt. Not a good thing, even for a street cat. As a lab scientist, Jess had learned all about parasites, and she identified it as a tape worm. It was time to take a step towards making this cat our cat. We had to find a good vet and get poor Jumbo some treatment. Our neighbors, who had a small indoor cat of their own, put us in touch with a mobile vet. The vet came out and gave Jumbo a shot to kill the worms.

> The Alleyway Freecycle. If you live in a city, placing anything in the alleyway ensures that it will be gone in minutes to hours, depending on its value and your neighborhood. I have unintentionally lost many items through the alleyway freecycle program, including saws and other tools I left outside for a few moments by mistake, and someone had driven by in an old truck, saw an opportunity, and ganked my stuff. This can be advantageous if you want to get rid of something quickly. Or if you see something you like. On a run around my neighborhood one day, I saw a cat tower that looked brand new, so I put it on my back and carried it home for Jumbo.

A funny finding from that encounter with the vet—she said the cat was not male, but female. She couldn't find the cat's penis. Jess thought this was hilarious. We had been assured the cat was male. Now, no penis. Female. Go figure. A few weeks before, I'd found an old cat tower through the "alleyway freecycle" and placed it on our front porch for Jumbo. After the worm shot, she holed up in the lookout of the tower and didn't come out for three days. I checked on her and, in what sounded like an onery British accent, she told me to "mind me own business if eh knew what wers best fer me." We thought the poor cat was dying or pregnant, as pregnancy was now a possibility, after all. On the fourth day, she strutted out good as new, well maybe not new, but not dying anymore. The worms were gone!

On December 2, Sierra completed the 50-miler in Arizona. The event went well. She took 3rd out of the females. Afterwards, she was tired and physically beat up, so she took four days off before returning to her training plan. I don't know what she did on those days. I hoped that she was resting, but knowing her, she was out kayaking or spearfishing.

Eight days after her race, I structured in a mock PT test to see where she was. That did not go well. She was still recovering from the race, it seemed. Her maxes were poor, and her 1.5 mile was at 12 minutes, a full 2 minutes slower than her initial test at the beginning of the season. This clearly illustrates the physical impact a 50-mile race can have on the body of even a seasoned ultrarunner. The post-race deleterious effects can last a long time. I knew she was faster than that, remembering one of my favorite lessons from Mike: fatigue masks performance. She was still fatigued from the race, so her true ability did not appear during the test. Now that the ultra was over, we could begin to put the pedal down and start accelerating her training towards a hypothetical mid-April rookie training start date. She was still waiting on a candidate offer.

A week after the slow 1.5-mile test, I had her run some broken 400-meter plus 200-meter intervals at a 6-minute mile pace, and she crushed them and said that she could have run faster. Relieved, I knew that we were still on track. She simply needed more time to recover. Her ultra had really set us back. The race was on December 2nd, and here we were on the 15th, and she was now feeling back to normal. We could have been training towards bolstering her PT tasks or working on hip stability during that time, but instead, she raced and recovered from racing.

At least Sierra was becoming a stronger hiker. During this month, I began to assign light pack hikes with exercises mixed into the middle. Here is a sample training session from the beginning of this month:

12/11	***Day 5 (Mon): Light Pack Hike + Exercises***		***Outcomes***	
W	General Warm-up			
	40 minute Light Pack Hike	35 lbs.		
	3 Rounds, of:		I hiked for a couple hours including the rounds at the top of the mountain. I ended up filling my pack up with rocks and found a great trail!	Perfect!!!
	Cut Line (or chop wood, or sledgehammer to tire)	2 minutes, hard effort		
	Lunges with Pack	16 reps		
	Burpees	8 reps		
	Squats with Pack	16 reps		
	40 minute Light Pack Hike	35 lbs.		
S	Complete Post-Workout Stretching & Foot Care!!!			

On this hike, she felt that her pack was too light, so she increased the pack's weight by placing in rocks as she worked her way up the trail. I thought this was clever.

Sometimes I would have a pack hike planned and she would go for a long run instead. While checking the spreadsheets and seeing that she didn't follow the program, I would immediately experience anxiety rise from my abdomen to my chest. It was difficult to predict what she would change and why. This was a common theme. She would do more reps or extra sets of exercises. She would train on rest days, sometimes performing large workloads of tasks that I had planned for her to complete the next day. This was problematic because the body needs rest between similar physical demands. What really blew my mind was that it seemed like she was continuing to get better despite following the program loosely. I wondered if she would improve faster if she followed the program to a "T." I maintained a soft grip on the reins here because, deep down, I felt at times that she knew what her body needed better than I did. This can be problematic in the long run though because athletes will almost always default to training what they are good at and will steer clear of their weaknesses.

To help improve our coaching relationship, I began to seek clarity from her when she missed a task or replaced a training session. Often, she would explain the switch was due to logistical reasons. Some days, she didn't have access to the specific equipment for a session, so she would hit her go-to, a long run. Other days, it seemed like she was simply listening to her body. The only problem with constantly listening to your body is that hers was geared towards running insanely long distances, and we still needed to induce a large shift to her muscle mass towards completing a ton of PT volume to withstand the onslaught she would face at rookie training. I felt like I was finally beginning to understand her better.

On December 18, Sierra was completing a 70-pound heavy pack hike for three miles and got a phone call from the Boise Smokejumper base during the task. She wrote, "I have no clue how I did this walk in 33:30 because Boise called during and I had an interview as I was pack testing!" Perhaps she was so excited to get this call that she pushed faster than she thought. The result was stellar. Eleven-minute miles with 70 pounds—that's quick! I asked her if she was considering Boise, and she said that she's seriously considering any base that offers her a job. I smiled wide when I read this text. Boise was the same base where Heidi went through rookie training. I secretly wanted Sierra to experience rookie training at Boise because I felt that it would be the toughest challenge for her. She seemed to seek tough challenges in her life to test herself. I didn't tell her how I felt because they didn't give her a candidate bid, yet, and I didn't want to impart my own desires onto Sierra. I was there to support and guide her training, not to influence her career path.

The rest of December rolled along. By the end of the month, Sierra's strict pull-ups went from 7 to 8. We were on pace for gaining one strict pull-up each month. This was good, but I thought we could do better. Her push-ups and sit-ups were also steadily improving, but I was concerned her rate of progress would not be enough to get her through rookie training. I hoped I was wrong.

For New Year's Eve, Jess was off this year, so we rented a Cabin in Big Bear and decided to invite some friends. We heated up some pizza in the oven, drank beer, played cards, and at midnight, toasted each other, the end of 2017, and the beginning of 2018, a year that seemed to hold promise for each of us. Jess loved San Diego already. She said she didn't miss Redlands at all, which silently stung. I was still seeking a solid foothold in San Diego. Jess had her job. I was starting from scratch, and it was more challenging than I had envisioned.

JANUARY 2018

The beginning of 2018 started out slow. I still lacked a brick-and-mortar job and spent most of my time growing an online training business from the oddly shaped office at the back of my little blue house. I began the process of recruiting personal training clients to train in the garage, and I continued to grow my online athlete group. When I had arrived in San Diego, I had a handful of athletes. Now, my roster was double that. Once or twice a month on the weekends when Jess worked, I still took the two-hour drive to train athletes in Redlands for extra cash and to visit friends. On the weekends when Jess was off, we walked on Coronado beach and talked about the wedding plans. I complained about Sierra's latest disregard for my training suggestions, and Jess would give her two cents, and I'd squint, nod quickly, throwing out uh-huhs, and clamp my mouth shut.

I was still acclimating to Jess working nights. Five nights a week, I was a bachelor. I wasn't lonely, but I was alone, often. My only friend was Jumbo. She seemed very unhappy. During "winter" in San Diego, it rained a bit and was "cold" sometimes, the temperature dipping into the 40s at night. Our hippie neighbors had renamed the cat Snowflake because she was completely white, and perhaps they thought it was funny because the name is so innocent, and she seemed so... grungy. Who knows? The name stuck.

In the evenings after a day of programming and feeling lost in the world of marketing for my business, when motivation to take another step towards a better future for myself dwindled, I put on a stocking cap, sat on the porch, and smoked a J. This was unusual behavior for me. My whole life, marijuana was not common. However, in my current predicament, feeling lost in San Diego, it seemed to calm my woes. Snow enjoyed a good buzz, too. I'd click my tongue twice and tap my lap, and the dirty white cat would glide over, jump smoothly up onto my thighs, and ask for a hit. I'd blow the smoke into her face, and she'd close her eyes, sniff it in, and purr away. We'd sit there together, enjoying our high in the crisp early evening as the final rays of sunlight faded into night. "Thanks for the hit, mate. Takes the edge right off." Yep, unmistakably British.

Sierra's 2018 training started out tough. Her heavy pack training weight on January 1st was 80 pounds for three miles. Up to this point, she had kept the pace between 33–35 minutes to complete this training task. Today, she finished in 47 minutes. This was a clear sign that the pack was now heavy to her, or so I thought until reading her feedback. She wrote, "We were so busy at work and i got 2 hours of sleep so I went into this pack test sleep deprived. I used my boots for the first time. I wore a 40 lb vest with 40 lbs. in a pck on top. the wieght was so uncomfortable on my shoulders!" After reading this, I thought that perhaps we could chalk up her slower, yet still plenty fast enough, time to sleep deprivation. Even a single night of decreased sleep can have a massive negative impact on mental and physical performance. Sierra's work caused her to experience this often.

The next day she also worked and had no time to complete her training. Instead of completing her strength training, she flew to Cedros Island off the Baha Peninsula of Mexico and went for a 6-mile run. The next five days she took off from training and spent her time freediving and spearfishing. She asked me to write her simple bodyweight training and short running workouts to help improve her 1.5-mile speed. She didn't get to any of these sessions. I had a feeling that she wouldn't, so I didn't let this bother me. Instead, I went back to the drawing board with her program. When an athlete takes time away from strength training, you can't start them back off where they were before the break. You must back off a bit. So, we did.

For Sierra's first training session back, she decided to combine two days of training into one, testing her pull-ups and realizing that she had lost only a single rep over her 6-day trip. That's not too bad. She also threw in an extra running session, completing a 4.5-mile run (which is very short for her), holding a 6:30-mile pace for 1.5 miles in the middle of this run. She wanted to prove to herself that she could run fast. It's funny how each athlete has their own individual tests that they deem important. I would have never asked her to perform this exact drill, but I'm glad that she did. It showed that she was getting faster, and that she could produce and hold decent running speed in the middle of a longer bout of running. This might come in handy at rookie training. I would not have had her test something like this until late February or early March. Apparently, she did gain some of her speed back already, and we had just over three more months for her to improve. I smiled and shook my head. Sometimes her audibles were good.

On January 10th, I scheduled Sierra to complete a light pack hike with 40 pounds, a mere 5 pounds heavier than last month's light pack training. She was at work on this day and couldn't get away for a long hike, so she strapped her pack on her back and hit the stair climber at the fire station for an hour, followed by a 15-minute circuit of sledgehammer strikes to a tire, lunges, squats, and burpees, all with her pack on. Another hour of stair climbing was scheduled, but she couldn't get to it. The station she worked at was very busy. They were called out that night and didn't sleep until the next day. This was a common event for Sierra, hitting a tough training session and following it up with little to no sleep, or the other way around.

Ever since Sierra got the call from Boise during her pack training, I had been throwing in extra pull-ups, push-ups and sit-ups to prepare her, mirroring what I had Heidi complete. The next training day was one of those days. Sierra started her training off with a 60-minute light pack training on the stair climber (yes, she'd decided to finish yesterday's workout. She's the type of person who doesn't like leaving loose ends). Then she maxed her strict pull-ups. Back up to 8 reps! Next, she completed a grueling workout containing hundreds of pull-ups, push-ups, sit-ups, and running. However, the work I asked her to do is still below what I thought she would need to be able to handle at rookie training. Could she do the full workload that day if I wrote it in? Yes, she could. But she shouldn't. Just because you can doesn't mean you should. This saying holds true in life and training. Her current maxes weren't high enough to handle the amount of volume without considerably breaking her down. In time, she would conquer the high volumes within a single workout. For now, I must help her move towards those standards.

She finished this wild training session with some stability work: glute bridges, walking lunges, and band pull-aparts, a shoulder stability drill. And comically, she skipped her cooldown stretching yet again. No amount of me pleading my case for warm-ups and cooldowns had gotten through to her.

The next day, Sierra was spent. Even after a full night's sleep, she could not complete her training. Instead, she hit her go-to and ran 7 miles. She also added that she had been going through extra stress because one of her friends had passed away.

Sierra: "I felt absolutley horrible this day! I jogged 7 miles because I couldn't get through the workout. I think I needed sleep and was exhausted from work and have been going through a lot of stress since one of my best friends died."

Me: "I am truly sorry to hear that, Sierra."

There it was. Poor Sierra was grieving, overworked, and now I was pushing her too hard. I felt guilty for adding stress to her life. I didn't verbally tell her, "Make sure that you do this training today, or else!" I simply wrote it in her spreadsheets, and she felt beholden to complete it. I should have known better.

By the middle of January, I wrote her a pack hike session over challenging terrain with elevation gain and loss. She loaded up 55 pounds and hit a really steep hill that she used to train on. Half-way through her hike at the 40-minute mark, I had her stop and complete a 20-minute AMRAP (As Many Rounds/Reps As Possible) of bodyweight and pack-loaded exercises, and cutting line. After completing this, she hiked back down. This was a challenging two-hour training session. I had written in an hour of light yoga to finish this training day, but she didn't have time. Instead, she ran three miles at sub-8:00/mile pace. The next day, I was ecstatic to see that she actually rested! I smiled, sighed, and shook my head in disbelief. She just might be rested enough to put up some good numbers on tomorrow's PT testing.

On the PT test, she completed a set of 9 pull-ups! A half month down, and an extra rep added to this task. She was now well on her way to her goal of 15 reps. Her push-ups today were not strong. She said that her arms were fatigued from the pull-ups. She crushed her sit-ups. To end this day's training, I wrote in another heavy pack training session. Since her last attempt at 80 pounds at the beginning of this month was tough, I kept the weight there to allow her body to adapt. This second attempt wasn't much better. We finally found Sierra's working weight. She complained that her pack was very uncomfortable. If she struggled with 80 pounds on her back, 110 pounds would bury her. We simply had to put in the time training this specific task. Sure, cardiovascular capacity is challenged here, and yes, the musculature of the feet, legs, and hips take a beating, but there are other important factors that get overlooked by those who have not rucked. Discomfort in the lower back can result from weakness in the abdominal muscles compared to the meaty back muscles (the lats, erectors, and quadratus lumborum), and the tissues and joints of the shoulders get sore from the shoulder straps of the pack pulling down with the entirety of the pack weight. Acclimating the body to these unique discomforts improves through sheer repetition and time. We were getting there. Sierra's mark this week was a blazing 50 minutes, leaving plenty of time to spare before the 65-minute Boise cutoff, or the 90-minute mark for Redding. I hoped that we could increase her strength over the next three months to handle the 30 extra pounds of pack weight.

To my surprise, the next day Sierra completed her foot care. I couldn't believe it! A few days before, she had taken a rest day and here she was today taking care of her feet. Even though she didn't have planter fasciitis like Heidi, with the amount of running and hiking miles that she put into her feet each week, foot care would go a long way to keeping her feet healthy, happy, and strong. As I looked through her spreadsheets, I poured myself a rye on the rocks with a splash of water. Jess laughed at me. She said that I was being silly for celebrating such small things. I half smiled, grumbled something, and took a swig. She was right. It was too early to celebrate anything, but it felt like these small things were leading to bigger wins.

Near the end of January, Sierra made use of more vacation. This time, she headed to Hawaii for two weeks. Even though she was on vacation, she liked to stay busy, so she asked me to write her bodyweight training and running workouts for each day except for a couple days where she would be spearfishing. She did a great job of completing the training I wrote for her. In addition, she went on a 9-mile run around Honolulu to explore the area, and she hit a 15-mile trail run at an easy pace. Sometimes, in the same day, she would spearfish. On January 21, 2018, she wrote, "Dove my ass off today!!!! Great workout. Good breath holds and pushed myself today diving 60 ft. and staying on the bottom for some time." Her lung capacity really was something special. The rest of her trip went well. We built bodyweight volume, accumulating tons of pull-ups, push-ups, and sit-ups at Hawaiian playgrounds. I wrote her only one rest day on this vacation, and she took that day to run 7 miles, hike 5 miles, and then swim for a while. She was like the energizer bunny. When she wasn't at work, she had more energy than anyone I had ever seen before. If only I could train her without the constraints of her firefighting job!

Jess and I had been in San Diego about three months now, and I was already getting stir-crazy spending every day at the house. Jess worked a lot, and I didn't know anyone in town. I was getting lonely. My only friend was that flea-filled alley cat. By now, I was spending most evenings with her on the porch, a glass of whiskey in one hand and a hand-rolled joint in the other. I'd tell her stories about Redlands, about life. She was a good listener, purring away in a pile on my lap, high as a kite, slurring British quips in here and there.

Professionally, it felt like I was losing some creativity in my training programs for Sierra and the other athletes I coached. I felt that picking up a part-time coaching position somewhere would help get my creativity flowing. The small handful of clients that I was coaching in my home gym wasn't enough. I'm a social person and gain energy from being around others, and this became even more apparent the longer I sat at home, alone. I found a sport-specific training facility and drove over to check it out. The place looked decent, and after reading business reviews and meeting the head coach, I applied for a part-time job.

Jessica was further settling in at the hospital. She was still a per-diem employee, so she took all the shifts that they offered. Her shift was PM, meaning that she would start at 5:00 p.m. and end at 1:30 a.m. This put her on a unique sleep schedule. She'd go to bed at 3:00 a.m. and wake at noon. Jess had not asked for me to get on her sleeping schedule, but I thought it would allow us to spend time together after she got home from work. I envisioned us watching a show together while eating popcorn at two in the morning. I tried to make it happen, but immediately I began to feel physically off from sleeping in so late, and I was alone after she left for work. My challenging transition to San Diego rolled onwards.

FEBRUARY 2018

Sierra got back to San Diego from Hawaii on February 1st. We now had about two and a half months left to prepare. I wasn't feeling confident that Sierra would be ready for rookie training. I was concerned that her PT volume and pack training exposure was too low. Logistically, we simply didn't have the training time each week. Sierra's full-time job was demanding of her time and energy. Many training sessions were a net neutral at best after working on a fire the evening before and sacrificing an entire night of sleep.

I knew how much the weighted carries mattered, so first on my list this month was the pack test. Sierra hadn't carried a heavy pack since before her Hawaii trip, which was more than two before, so I started her out lighter than where we left off in the middle of January, working at 75 pounds instead of 80. When reading her feedback for the heavy pack carry, I found some great news casually camouflaged into the spreadsheets. She wrote, "I did this walk with my dad because I thought it might ease the pain! Lol we talked the whole time and I decided to take it easy since I'm going to Redding and need to do the test in 90 minutes. Today I did 50 minutes with not too much pain! It helped having my dad to talk to." Sierra got a rookie candidate bid from Redding. Finally!!! And she didn't even think to tell me.

Later in this same training day, she went off script and went on an 11-mile run, also with her dad. Then going further off the plan, she completed a total of 50 pull-ups. I had planned for her to test pull-ups tomorrow, so in my feedback, I wrote, "Hopefully this extra gymnastic work doesn't decrease your training outcomes tomorrow."

It turned out that her extra work did negatively impact the next day's training, but only in the pull-ups (luckily). Sierra was continuing to learn the same lessons. This time, she admitted fault in the comments by stating, "You were right." I was relieved to see that I was getting through to her, albeit slowly. There was still time to improve our communication. Why did those 50 reps that she had completed the day before hinder her max reps today? As an athlete, if you want to perform well tomorrow, you can't train today with a high number of total repetitions or sets with a high number of reps compared to your max reps without experiencing fatigue and decreased performance in those specific tasks tomorrow. That's why completing high workloads in rookie training can negatively impact PT scores after the first day.

Sierra's push-ups and sit-ups went well because she had rested those tasks for the last few days. On a slightly more positive note, I was happy to see that she completed her foot care after this session. Her feedback, as had been the case for our entire relationship thus far, surprised me. "We played frisbee in the morning and I ran 3.5 miles during frisbee and did 150 air squats so my legs were tired, but I don't know why my pull-ups sucked so bad." I knew that optimal results are produced from quality training, not fatigued training, and I explained this. She was bound to get it soon. My head was constantly sore now from banging it against my desk.

After a long day of programming and slogging through blind and dumb to business marketing strategies, I would go out on the porch and sit with Snowflake, and we'd commiserate. "Alright?" she'd ask. "You know, busy, bored, having a tough time down here," I'd answer. She'd ask for a hit, and I'd give her what she wanted. Today we passed the time in silence.

This is a great time to talk about optimal training versus hard training. I have written extensively so far about the extreme physical demands of rookie training. Testing and passing the PT standards (pull-ups, push-ups, and sit-ups) is important to the rookie trainers. If a rookie fails to meet or exceed the minimum standards, no matter how fatigued, they are washed from the program immediately. Athletes must be mentally and physically ready to battle unique combinations of stressors and fatigued PT tests.

Occasionally, training this way is helpful. However, constantly aligning training circumstances to test athletes when fatigued (after long bouts of running, etc.), physically limited (adding external resistance to make a regular task harder, like those oxygen-restriction breathing masks), or in a sleep debt is sub-optimal. We don't adapt well from the stressors of life with insufficient sleep. The stimulating dose of stress must be just beyond our current level of ability. Therefore, the mechanisms that drive performance are never fully stimulated through sub-optimal conditions, even if the mental training gleaned from the experience is top-notch. Therefore, when undergoing hard training, the coach and athlete assume the risk and hope for the best. You roll the dice.

Any coach can make training hard if they try. In a single training session, simply push an athlete right up to the edge of their current strength, endurance, or skill capacity and hold them there for a long time. This will be hard in many ways. Sleep depriving an athlete and then completing a normal training session is hard. Running an athlete for a few hours and then testing their benchmarks is hard. However, this will never yield optimal adaptations. And this fact matters. A lot. There is something to be said for making sure that you sprinkle some servings of "hard" training in to ensure the athlete has grit, but make sure the dose is worth the risk. Hard training is risky.

In my opinion, the best way to prepare an athlete for unknowable testing parameters is to train optimally ***most*** of the time. This means spending most of the preparation time garnering maximum adaptations to create an athlete that is as strong and fast and anti-fragile as possible at the start of rookie training.

In the middle of February, I began to feel that I could more clearly predict Sierra's changes to my programming and planning. As my predictions improved, I felt better about the whole process. Furthermore, having Redding as our target boosted my confidence because the standards are lower than at Boise. I'm not sure how Sierra felt about the lower PT standards, but I imagined it took some pressure off her. The pack test would be easier with a longer time cap, too. Even though she loved to challenge herself, I think she knew we were cutting it close.

I felt that we were beginning to bond through the spreadsheets. During a three-part light pack hike with exercises mixed in, I loved Sierra's feedback. "I hiked up a steep bluff from my boat in Baja and it took 40 minutes to get to the top. Did the circuit at the top, then hiked for another 25 minutes and did another circuit, then hiked down. Ended up being 5.3 miles and 1:45 for time. It was beautiful and my dad came with me. Then we ran 6 miles on the beach.

Great workout!" I responded with, "That sounds like a nice time. Does your dad do the workouts with you? Good job here!!!" And she responded, "Lol no way! My dad sat down and enjoyed the view. He did 4 squats!!" I laughed to myself. It felt like we were finding our groove. She finished this training session with barefoot weird walks on the beach.

Weird walks. I learned these from Mike. I first saw him instruct his jumpers to perform them in a sand volleyball court in March once the rough midwestern winter died down. There were four main variations: 1) walking up on the balls of the feet, 2) walking on the heels, 3) walking on the inner arches, and 4) walking on the outer arches. Mike called these barefoot walks, but the athletes complained that they were weird, so I renamed them "weird walks." The idea is to strengthen the muscles of the feet and lower legs.

Up until this point, each training day was a single modality, a long pack hike with exercises, or a day in the gym strength training, or a long run followed by a quick PT session. It was now time to ramp training up. Sierra had several days off in a row before she started back up at work, so I was determined to give her a packed stretch of training. For the next four days, I loaded her up with multiple three-a-days. And for the first time in any of her training sheets, I urged her to take a rest and eat between each individual training session. I wrote this in **BOLD** purple and white, clear as day. Even though the quantity of training was high, I wanted the quality to remain high as well. Getting specific with when and how to rest is one way to help enforce quality. Here is the breakdown for this stretch of training:

- **Day one**—Running Intervals (6 x 400 meters with short rest), a 2-hour trail run, and yoga
    - She completed the 400's at 5:40 mile pace, which is fast for an endurance specialist, then went on a twenty-mile trail run. She skipped the yoga because she ran an hour longer than I had written her and ran out of time. The reason that she ran for an extra hour? She writes, "Ok I did 3 hours ... had to switch this workout with Saturday's because I had a trail running partner ... we did 16 miles at Daley Ranch. Great run! Except I did this before the intervals." I couldn't believe that she had run 16 miles and then had done her 5:40-paced intervals. That's crazy. I was concerned that she had started this four-day block of training with too much gusto.

- **Day two**—PT test, a medium pack hike, and yoga
    - I wanted to PT test her today after her heavy running yesterday. Her pull-ups were at 7 (good enough), push-ups at 33 (her worst test of the year), and sit-ups at 90 (not bad). These numbers would fly at Redding. She came through the 1.5-mile in 10:00, which is also good enough. I was happy with her fatigued results and let her know. After a break, she hiked at Del Rosa with the hotshots and her pack was heavier than I had

planned. She was so exhausted from her fatigue from yesterday and now the heavier-than-planned pack that she skipped the mid-hike exercises that I wrote in for her.

- **Day three**—Intervals followed by a power and strength training session
    - She attempted more running intervals today, but it didn't go well. She felt very tired after a single round of an 800-meter followed by two 400-meter runs, then quit. She then swam a mile afterwards, which felt good. I dug into her today, writing, "From one workout day where you ran 1 hour too long, and performed the intervals out of order, you were wrecked for a few days. To be successful in rookie training, you must be able to overcome setbacks like this. The way to teach your body to combat adversity is to train as hard as you HAVE TO, but not an ounce harder. If you train out of order, it robs you of capacity in later training. If you run too far, it takes from future workouts and does not give you much in return. Every day counts. Every set, rep. It will all matter in Redding. Please keep that in mind when you complete the rest of your training over the next two months!!!" I had been holding that in for a while now. It felt good to get my feelings off my chest, and I hoped that I came off as compassionate. Sierra did not respond in writing, but I know she read it.
    - After a rest and some food, she hit her third training session for the day, the power and strength. She surprised herself here and, "actually felt good with the weights—weird." I agreed. That was unexpected. I was glad that she got some quality work in on this day, even if much of her training fell apart at the seams. The strength session was my last scheduled training for her on this day, but she decided to end with one additional session—some yoga.
- **Day four**—Heavy PT volume, a long pack hike, and yoga
    - This day was my toughest yet. I knew that she worked the next day, and this was the fourth day in a row of training. I wanted to push Sierra to see what she could do and how she would recover from this short and intense "shock" cycle. Today's training started off with hundreds of reps of pull-ups, push-ups, sit-ups, and running, combined in a circuit. She completed all the pull-ups and push-ups in unbroken sets, which is a big win in a heavily fatigued state. After a rest and some food, I wrote in a light pack hike with 35 pounds, again keeping her weight milder, but I programmed her a three-hour push with bodyweight exercises mixed in. Instead of hiking, Sierra completed this on the stair climber and completed all the other work! She finished this session with yoga. She writes, "this was a killer day!!!!" And I agreed. From here on, most of her training would be two-a-days, and sometimes three-a-days. She made it through, ready for more.

After a day of rest, Sierra was back at it. That single day of rest worked wonders for her running, but her pull-ups and push-ups were still fatigued from the previous week. That made perfect sense. Her running capacity was massive in comparison to her training age for the PT tasks. Of course, her running recovered more quickly. Two days later, she hit some fast 800-meter intervals and shortened my specified rest from 3:00 of complete rest to 1:30 with a 12-minute mile jog instead. This was a massive change to the intended stimulus of the workout. Instead of taking the full duration of complete do-nothing-with-your-body rest, she cut the rest duration in half and ran slowly instead of doing nothing. When I saw her feedback in the spreadsheet, I laughed out loud while shaking my head. Leave it to Sierra to make training harder almost every time.

For her mid-month heavy pack training, I had suggested she attempt three miles with 85 pounds, and she loaded it to 90 and again walked with her dad. She came through in 55 minutes and didn't push herself too hard, she said. With the Redding standard set at completing this carry in 90 minutes, she still had plenty of padding. And the fact that she didn't need to push very hard to maintain this pace was reassuring. Maybe we weren't that far off after all.

A day later, she was training at her Forest Falls cabin and set a personal best time on the Vivian Creek Trail. She had run this route earlier in training and took it all the way up to the top of San Gorgonio. She followed my strict 2-hour training duration on this trail run and turned around an hour in, getting back in time to make the cutoff. Sierra was proud of herself, writing, "Hit a PR on this run. I did 8 miles rt and went up Vivian creek and ran the whole thing. I've always had to walk the first sections of that trail!!! Great run!!" I was blown away by her ability to push herself despite the heavy training volume that I was putting her through. This trail run was after a 90-minute strength and power training session.

After this training day, I wrote her another PT-focused session followed by more intervals. This time, 8 rounds of 200-meters at a fast pace with lots of rest. I wanted to help push her speed! The next two training days were highlighted in orange. Both read, "Full rest day." She responded, "Now how am I going to take 2 rest days??!!!!!!! 😮 🤪 im gonna go crazy." I laughed and told her she'd get through it. She didn't write any feedback in, so either she actually did rest on those days, or she trained and didn't tell me about it.

After those rest days, we both expected her PT marks to increase. She had put in a ton of work this month. Her pull-ups crept back up to 8, but she felt like she could squeeze out 9 or 10 reps if fully recovered. Her push-ups went well, and she completely smoked her sit-ups. I had been training her sit-ups this month using on-the-minute intervals. We started out with higher volume, 8 sets of 25 reps on the minute for a total of 200 reps and moved to 6 sets of 30 reps on the minute (180 reps). On this testing day, instead of asking her to collect a max set of reps in 3 minutes, I had her complete 45 seconds of max reps with 15 seconds of rest, for three rounds. She completed 40, 40, and 39 reps for a total of 119 reps in 2:45. She had just smashed her old 3-minute PR with fifteen seconds to spare! Finally, we could check off one of her PT tasks as damn-good enough. I actually jumped out of my chair when I read her results, fist pumped, and yelled, "There we go!" I then looked around and remembered that Jess was at work; it was Wednesday, and I was alone. It still felt good! We were doing it!

By now, it was the middle of ski season and Sierra flew to Colorado. In addition to all the other physical challenges that Sierra did, of course, she also skied. Once again, her feedback blew me away. "Skied again today ... just did 3 hours yesterday and another 3 today but today I hiked up to 12,000 ft and skied deep powder since it snowed and my legs were burning !!"

This ski trip, and all other scheduling concerns, had been alleviated through Sierra and me using a shared tab in the spreadsheets called, "Specific Planning." Each line was a day, and I had a place for her to put where she was here staying and what she had planned. Without it, I don't think we would have made it this far. Since she was in Colorado for five and a half days and the weather didn't permit running outside, I exclusively programmed gym workouts. Or so I thought. Once again, her feedback knocked me. "Ran 11 miles, about 2 hours because I was exploring new trails and ended up way outside of town ... it was about 15 degrees and winds up to 30 mph and 9,000 ft so I was pushing it. Exhausted !!!!!" And I thought she wouldn't be running. My mistake. Of course, she would run.

The next day, she rested and traveled back to San Diego. She had few workdays coming up. The day after she got home, I scheduled another heavy pack training, this time with 100 pounds. She completed this one plenty fast, writing, "53:06 ... I sped up on the last mile. Probably could have gone a little faster but I think this time is just fine with 37 minutes to spare for the test. I'm confident that I can get the same time or faster with another 10 lb. definitely an uncomfortable 53 minutes though!"

On the last day of February, I wrote her a PT-specific session with some nasty combinations:

- Complete a set of max pull-ups and rest 60 seconds between. Keep going until you can only perform a single rep. Stop, rest 3 minutes, and repeat for three total rounds. She completed 108 total pull-ups here.
- For push-ups and sit-ups, I instructed her to complete 12 rounds, resting 30–40 seconds between each task, of 10 push-ups (120 total reps) and 20 sit-ups (240 total reps). She said this was easy.

This month was fantastic. Despite all the traveling, work, multiple living locations, and her vacation, it felt like we were connecting well. I felt like I understood her now, and it seemed that she was starting to trust me. I felt all warm and fuzzy about how things were going. In the meantime, between watching over Sierra's spreadsheets and programming on odd days to fit her schedule, I was enjoying my new job at the sport-specific training facility. It was a challenging switch from my previous coaching experience. I spent most of that time teaching movement mechanics to adolescents. I taught them sprinting, hopping, jumping, medicine ball throws, change of direction, and general strength training principles. The toughest part was corralling them and holding their attention. The youngest teams were eight-year-olds, but they weren't necessarily the toughest. Some of the thirteen-year-olds were the moodiest and least responsive humans I had ever coached. It was eye opening.

I coached from 2–8 p.m. Monday through Friday. Jess would have to get used to me being out of the house. Before my new job, we had gotten into a routine after 4 p.m. I'd help her pack lunch and kiss her goodbye, knowing the next time I would see her was close to 2 a.m., and I'd be sound asleep. That routine was now disappearing. I would miss it.

At home, Jess and I were putting the finishing touches on our wedding plans. We sent out the invites in January and the RSVPs were rolling in. The year before in May, when Heidi was still in rookie training, we found a wonderful location in Oak Glen, a small town less than an hour's drive east of Redlands. Located up a narrow winding road through the foothills of the San Bernardino mountains, the venue was on a hillside, complete with a barn, a vineyard, and a pond. We had scheduled a few other places for viewing, but I had a strong feeling that this was going to be the location. When we first arrived, Jess immediately teared up. I knew then we would be married there.

MARCH 2018

Our wedding was scheduled for two months from now in early May. Both of our families lived in Illinois, along with all of Jessica's high school and college friends. My high school friends were in Arizona. It would be a destination wedding for everyone on the guest list except for most of my college buddies who were living around the Redlands area. Wedding preparations were in full swing. Jess was working full time and sometimes overtime shifts at the lab, so for planning the wedding, we had leaned into minimalism which considerably decreased the number of decisions.

Aside from wedding planning, we didn't spend too much time together. Jess had recently picked up a part-time, noc-shift position in addition to her full-time gig. On one of Jess's rare full weekends off, we drove up to Redlands to cake taste, visit the florist, and see the venue one last time before the wedding rehearsal two days before our wedding. I ate my fill of cake. Jess laughed at me and called me a little fatty. I shrugged with a smile mid chew and shoved more cake in my mouth. The baker did say to eat as much as we wanted.

Sierra and I were gearing up for her most challenging training block. We were now six and a half weeks away from rookie training at Redding. I planned to peak her training volume 5 weeks out, which was only a week and a half away. She was training 6 days a week now, between 3 and 4 hours a day, sometimes 5. In the weeks to come, we shifted into another gear.

Sierra had just finished one of her grad school classes on March 6 and wrote in the spreadsheets, "Really crappy week for me!! Sitting at the computer stressed and mayor lack of sleep ... fortunately I passed my class so I can totally focus on training!!!!" I was glad to hear that. She sounded ready to tackle the insane volume that I had planned for her.

After months of getting to know one another, we began to step in stride. On phone calls, Sierra now seemed bubbly and excited to move forwards. We had come a long way from that first phone call and our initial awkward training session in my old garage.

Sierra's final preparation weeks were filled with more running, long hikes carrying heavy packs with exercises mixed in, plenty of high-volume PT prep, and other miscellaneous conditioning tasks she might encounter in rookie training to inoculate her from the soreness that she might experience if she didn't receive exposure beforehand. Soreness during rookie training is inevitable, but if we could cut it down even a little bit, that would make her journey that much less painful. Heck, she might even pass.

She was now rucking with 55–60 pounds on three-plus hour hikes up sleep grades and stopping mid hike to complete a circuit containing a laundry list of exercises like bodyweight squats, lunges, burpees, and core work, and loaded exercises like deadlifts and squats using her pack as resistance.

Unexpectedly, about a third of the way into the month, on the last training day before her official volume peak week, she set a personal best of 9 pull-ups. I did not ask her to test that day because I had planned a full PT test four days later, where she could only squeeze out 8 reps. This is about the time I realized that she was testing her max pull-ups almost daily. This is not good. Frequently testing one's body to the max, even with a single exercise like pull-ups, is risky for the muscles and joints involved, and it's not great on the psyche, either. Over time, this can place an unusually large psychological burden upon each testing bout and decreases the effectiveness of normal volume training by constantly fatiguing the athlete. When you are testing, you aren't training. You are revealing performance potential, which is taxing and risky.

During the PT test in her peak week, she also completed 55 push-ups and 120 sit-ups. Each of these marks were personal bests. She also set a season PR in the 1.5-mile at 9:33. I was proud of this PT test, especially during her peak week where her body was well on its way to a severe physical beatdown from the training load. However, she was upset with her PT score. She wrote, "This pack test felt horrible! I finished the 2 miles but had to stop and rearrange my pack so I didn't time it. Then I was upset about my pull-ups and had a total emotional breakdown!" There it was. She had let her pull-up performance dictate how she performed in her pack test. She had finally revealed her center. Her weak point. This was exactly what we must address before she arrived at rookie training.

I wrote a response to her:

Beyond passing your necessary score of 7 reps here, so that's good. There are a few possible explanations why you pulled 8 reps here and not 9 or more. 1) you were 1 day of rest too much. I think this explanation is unlikely. 2) You could still be fatigued from your max set 3 days ago on 3/11. This is more likely. If you use it all, you lose it for about 5–7 days. After that recovery period, you will adapt and get a little bit better. 3) The testing format stresses you out, you put too much pressure on yourself on the pull-ups, and cave under the pressure. I don't know if this is what you experienced. You can think it through and let me know. IF this is the case, DO let me know. We have time to work on testing anxiety. No Joke.

It also didn't help that she had been working the night before at the fire station and only had about four hours of sleep. In hindsight, this was most likely the main reason that she put up lower numbers than expected. That, and the added accumulation of fatigue from the peak week. Physical and mental fatigue cause our emotions to run haywire. That is part of the beauty of rookie training. The rookie trainers creatively and brutally push the rookies to the edge to expose their true selves. Once they are exposed, the rookie trainers can clearly see who would make a good smokejumper, and who would be a liability to the team or themselves.

Late that night while reading Sierra's training notes, I wrote back to her:

The nature of the PT Test, and all of smokejumper rookie training is to find and expose your weaknesses. They want to know three very important things: 1) Are you PHYSICALLY FIT to withstand the demands of THE JOB you are testing to partake in? 2) Are you MENTALLY FIT to withstand those job demands? And 3) How bad do you want it? That's it. If you are not physically fit, you will not make it through. I know that you ARE physically fit enough to make it through. If you are physically fit enough, but not mentally fit, then you will not make it through. If you are physically and mentally fit to make it through, but don't want it bad enough, they will see this, they will press that button, and they will make you quit. All of the training that you have undergone so far is to prepare you for what you will experience in a month. Do not let your pull-ups cause you an emotional breakdown! Use that experience as a way to catapult yourself further, positively. If the rookie trainers sense you down on yourself, they will pounce on you until you quit. The reason they seek to find ANY weakness is because it is a matter of life and death. They don't want anyone to pass through who could be a liability. I know you can do this. I think you do, too. So, you must remain stoic. Don't let them see you mentally broken or maimed, no matter what. Keep your head up. Call me tomorrow if you need to talk.

For the rest of March, Sierra kept her head up, worked hard, wrote solid feedback into the spreadsheets, and completed over 90% of what I asked her to do. She had to complete some tasks and days out of order because of work conflicts, but she got it done. We had made it through the volume peak without any injuries. Her body had held up beautifully. Her mind had broken just a little, which I was happy about because now that her mental "Achilles heel" was exposed, we could work on bolstering her before Redding, which was now less than three weeks away.

APRIL 2018

My wedding was a month out. My guts were tossing and turning around in my belly. There was still so much to do. Jess and I were putting the finishing touches on the guest list and scheduling the wedding rehearsal and rehearsal dinner. We had a laundry list of wedding details to button up. I wasn't sleeping well, and my temper coaching the kids was disintegrating. One night after Jess left for work, I went out on the porch to get some fresh air and was met by Snowflake, who hopped up on my lap. Even she noticed my stress. "Aren't you proper miffed?" she asked. "Yes," I responded. I couldn't hide anything from her.

Jess was still working full time at the hospital and the part-time job was tacking extra days onto her work life. Sometimes she'd work 12 days in a row. To pass the time, I stayed busy with the athlete training center and taking care of my online programming clients. My athlete list was growing larger still. I was at a dozen athletes, having picked up two nutrition clients. Heidi was on my athlete list again this year, but not in preparation for rookie training. She was now a smokejumper. At the beginning of each season, returning smokejumpers must show up and undergo a PT test to ensure they are physically fit for the upcoming season. Heidi's goal this time around was a perfect score on the PT test. 400 points.

About a month out from the wedding, my best friend, CC, and my younger brother, Andy, threw me a bachelor party. They rented a large house in La Jolla, a ritzy sea town just north of the city of San Diego and invited all my old college friends. The weekend was a lovely mess. It started out civilized that first afternoon, but shortly after everyone arrived, we started the party and didn't stop. Don't worry, Jessica had her fun as well with a bachelorette party back in Chicago! I imagine hers was just as wild.

The Sunday afterwards, we cleaned up the house and, surprisingly, got out before 11 a.m. I grabbed some greasy hangover-fixing food with Andy, CC, and a few others before heading home to resume my life as husband-to-be and online coach. Programming for Sierra and the rest of my crew that day was a challenge. My brain was toast, and it took me eight hours to complete what I could usually finish in five. Luckily, Sierra's preparation for Redding was almost over. She was already a week into her taper. What could go wrong?

Sierra had made it through the toughest training block. It was now time to reveal her true ability. On the top right of the spreadsheet comment box, highlighted in yellow and in bold, I warned Sierra, **"DO NOT do extra work today. Stick to the sets and reps. This workout is meant to be easy. The purpose is to develop a habit of easy training before your PT test. Routines ensure success by making success part of a routine."**

I thought she might respond with some quip about doing extra work anyway, but she wrote about sleep deprivation instead. "Completed workout and did no extra. I got virtually no sleep the last 2 nights at work. This 72 hour shift was a killer. Did hoselays today and large ladders yesterday. Vehicle fire today. In and out of turnouts the last two shifts. Exhausted !!" I was concerned that her job was going to ruin the perfect taper that I had in mind for her. She was working really hard, and her sleep was suffering. The past few weeks and the three upcoming are arguably the most crucial for demands on the body and mind, and sleep deprivation is destructive to everything, including recovery, performance, and mental clarity.

Despite the stress from work, she seemed to experience the effects from the taper rather quickly. A few days into taper week one, she wrote, "So weird! I ran so fast today and felt great??? I ran my warm-up mile and then ran the 3 middle miles in 20:30 without trying that hard ... then my cool down in 8 minutes." In the middle of a 5-mile run, Sierra completed the middle three miles at 6:50 per mile pace. I was happy with this result, and Sierra was positively surprised. However, I knew this was just the beginning of the performance improvements which she would experience over the next 20 days before rookie training began. Heidi's supercompensation was massive and had lasted over three weeks from the end of her taper. I hoped that Sierra's would also have a long slow burn.

> Supercompensation in physical training refers to the temporary performance enhancement that occurs after a period of training and recovery where the body surpasses it's pre-trained capabilities.

However, a few days later, Sierra could only squeeze out 6 pull-ups and failed to complete a sit-up workout that I thought she would crush. I asked her if she was fatigued, and she replied that she just needed sleep. Work was still running her hard. Fortunately, she was planning to attend a conference the next day, followed by several days off work. She used this time to catch up on sleep. After resting from training the day of the conference, on the next day, after only a single day of rest, Sierra crushed a heavy pack test. She wrote, "46:40! I'm happy because I finally feel some improvement ! I started out with a 17 minute mile and then just kept speeding up almost to a jog. I'm so surprised but I felt really strong!!! 😊" This was her heaviest and fastest heavy pack training yet, and all she needed was one rest day and two back-to-back nights of complete sleep.

With less than two weeks left, Sierra took one last trip to recharge with some spearfishing off her kayak in Baja, Mexico. She continued to train and followed my taper plan. She posted some great PT numbers one day and was scheduled to rest the next day, but instead of resting, she went for a "light 6-mile run." Frustrated, I wrote to her that this was a bad idea. I knew the next day was a hard running workout. Sure enough, the next day, Sierra wrote in her feedback, "Completed the first mile and then I couldn't hold the pace for the second mile during the last quarter mile. I don't know why my legs felt so bad?!" My temper flared. On the verge of yelling through the keyboard, I responded, "You ran 6 miles yesterday on your rest day. I am tired of telling you to rest on your rest days. You ruin future workouts when you work on days you should be resting. Less is more, especially in these last two weeks. More is not better. Please believe and trust me on this. You do not have time to waste on junk volume. EVERY METER COUNTS. EVERY REP COUNTS."

Sierra: "Yes I know ... I just thought that the jog was nothing. Maybe it does take a toll"

Me: "Not maybe. It does. Right now more than ever, rest is your best weapon!"

All those insecurities and doubts that I had pushed down deep before coaching Sierra came rushing back and hit me with full force, plus interest. A gaping pit gave way in my stomach. Sierra's cavalier nature of going off-script, plus the pressure of the wedding, and my own lack of self-content in working at the athlete training center hit me. I slumped over the desk with my head in my hands and dug my fingers into the back of my neck. I stayed there a while, attempting to push the emotions back down.

Sierra: "I had a death in my immediate family totally unexpected so I'm trying to power through but honestly having a tough time."

The next day, with one week to go, someone close to Sierra had passed away. I found out through the spreadsheets, and when I read this, my jaw dropped. I could not believe the timing. I sent her my condolences and wondered what was going to happen. Her training for the next few days was spotty. She just couldn't muster up the energy. I was worried about her, so I called her to talk. She sounded okay and said she was fine, just grieving. Fine is never a word I want to hear, especially one week out from the most demanding physical challenge of her career.

My heart ached for her. Sierra was grieving and seemed to have given up on her training, at least momentarily. She took the rest of the week off from the San Diego Fire Station for bereavement leave and drove up to Redding on Thursday. Rookie training was set to begin the following Monday. I wished her luck. After months of broken training and through a fog of sadness, rookie training day one had arrived. I held onto a thread of hope.

MAY 2018

Sierra's situation had intensified significantly. When she arrived at Redding for rookie training, after two weeks of physical training and testing to ensure the rookies could physically hack it, the rookie trainers decided to take the group to train in Boise for week three. What?! She said all the smokejumper bases were transitioning from round to square Ram Air parachutes in the next year or two, and Redding had elected to make the change this season. The rookie trainers at Redding did not know how to teach the Ram Airs because they had been using the rounds for decades. Boise offered to train them. So off to Boise Sierra went, along with her fellow rookie smokejumpers and rookie trainers so they could all learn on the squares together. I couldn't believe it. Sierra was headed to Boise after all, the same place that Heidi had undergone rookie training. I was just happy to hear she'd made it through the first two weeks. From my limited understanding of the timeline, the initial weeks are heavily loaded with grueling physical demands meant to test and break the candidates who are physically unqualified. Apparently, Sierra could handle the physical demands, which was reassuring. However, the next week at Boise, week three, would be highly technical, and the weeks after that would continue to increase in complexity. I hoped that she was ready.

The wedding week was upon us. While Jess and I were making final preparations, Sierra was at rookie training. Even though I was thoroughly enveloped in all things wedding, Sierra was still on my mind. At random times throughout the week, I wondered what she was suffering through, and if she was performing like we'd hoped. She had just endured 5 months of intense training, more than she ever had before, and the bulk of it was time spent improving physical skills that she really didn't enjoy working on all that much. All the while, she had been completing a second master's degree, working full-time, and taking a handful of vacations which she trained through. She had her cake and ate it too, it seemed. Along the way, a close friend of hers had passed away. And within the last week before rookie training began, an immediate family member had passed away. That was a lot of life within a short stretch. I mentally sent her strength.

Two days before the wedding, the venue called Jess and me and asked one last time if we wanted to pay a bunch of extra money to put up a tent over the reception area. It had been raining at the venue for a few days, and the temperature was California-chilly, hovering below 60 degrees. We looked at the forecast and rolled the dice. No tent, save the money. Plus, the tent would obscure a breathtaking view of the canyon and mountains. We had many guests coming from the Midwest and wanted them to get the full Southern California experience. No tent.

The day before the wedding, we drove up from San Diego with our car fully packed with everything we needed. Decorations, wedding attendee gifts, alcohol (it was a bring your own booze location), Jess's dress, my tuxedo, and of course, the rings, or so I thought. We arrived at the venue with umbrellas and thick raincoats for the rehearsal. It was cold and rainy. The venue again asked if we wanted a tent for tomorrow for twice the price as the previous day's quote. No thank you, we said, letting our bet ride one final time. The rehearsal went off without a hitch despite the weather, and afterwards, we went to dinner in downtown Redlands, offering our parents, who had never met, a chance to get to know each other.

WEDDING DAY

The night before, we had stayed at a Native American casino about 20 minutes from the venue. Per tradition and superstition, Jess and I slept in separate rooms. I was not to see her again until she walked down the aisle with her father. I slept in late, knowing that my process to get ready for the wedding was short. Shower, dress, hair. That's it. Piece of cake. While showering, I had a random thought shoot through my head. Did I pack the rings? After drying off, with my pulse elevating, I put on some run-around clothes and jogged down to the car in the parking garage, trying to keep from panicking. I dug through the boxes in the trunk, in the back seat. No rings in sight. Time to freak out. I started sweating despite the chilly morning air. I sat in the passenger seat of my old Malibu and contemplated what to do. There was time to drive down to San Diego and back before the wedding. It could take less than 4 hours if I drove like a banshee. I could do so without even telling Jess. I should not tell her. She would freak out. But then another thought occurred. The casino had a gift shop, complete with jewelry. I went in and bought two rings, immediately relieved. I also relished the thought of Jess's confusion at the alter when I placed a different ring on her finger than the ones we had purchased together. Jess and I often teased each other, but a prank like this was a big step up. A sly smile crossed my lips.

On our seventh anniversary, in front of our closest friends and family, Jess and I declared our love for each other, promised to care for each other until death, and were married. I did surprise Jess with the switched rings at the alter and that got a good laugh from our guests as a wave of understanding swept through the crowd. Not to be outdone, Jess developed a plan to even the score later that evening.

When I was an impressionable young lad attending a cousin's wedding, during the garter dance, the groom reappeared from under his wife's dress with the garter belt in his mouth. I was shocked and impressed. One of my onlooking older cousins near me yelled out, "You're not a man unless you take the garter belt off with your teeth!" And to that day, I believed it to be true.

For the past month, I had been working each night on a choreographed dance routine to remove Jess's garter belt. After thirty years since learning about garter belts and manhood, my time had come. I chose the song, "Mississippi Queen," and at the end of my dance number, I ripped my shirt off sending buttons everywhere as everyone in attendance gasped in surprise, and I crawled across the dance floor on my bare stomach, making my way under the unfurling fabric of her big cream-colored dress. I spent an unusual amount of time—what felt like an eternity—under that dress. Confusion set in. The garter belt was nowhere to be found. I took my head out and peeked at Jess, who by now was laughing hysterically. She pulled the garter belt out from between her brazier and dropped it on my bare chest as I lay on my back looking up at her. The crowd went wild! To this day, I still seek my manhood.

The next week, Jess and I went to Hawaii on our honeymoon. Jess has a rule when we go on vacation—no work. That's easy for her. When she clocks out, her job is done. There is nothing for her to bring home from the hospital. However, I'm in a different boat. As a coach, I am openly available to my athletes, especially when one of them is in the middle of rookie training! While sitting on a beach in Maui, as Jess took a nap, it felt like a safe time for me to sneak check-in texts to Sierra. Sierra was out in the wilderness finishing up her third week of smokejumper rookie training. After a brutal first week, she had set personal best marks in the PT test. I was proud! The taper seemed to work nearly as well for Sierra as it had for Heidi.

At the end of week three, my phone rang. I was preparing dinner, grilling chicken breasts on the roof of our hotel in Hawaii. Jess was back in the room making a salad, so I thought it was her calling to ask me something. It wasn't. Sierra was calling. What could she be calling about? At the end of each past week, she had texted me how rookie training had gone. Something was wrong. I answered and immediately knew that the news was bad. Sierra solemnly told me that she had washed out at Boise. She had trouble with the jump protocols, and that was enough. She was unfit for smokejumping. They said she had done well with the PT testing and heavy pack tests, but that wasn't enough. She seemed numb. I thanked her for letting me know and ended the call. I had also burnt the chicken. I slumped my shoulders, hung my head, and brought the charred chicken breasts back to the room. I told Jess about Sierra over dinner. She gave me a hug and said that I had tried my best.

We did all that we could have done with the given constraints. A wave of negative thoughts and emotions began to swirl within me. I hadn't driven her hard enough. I should have insisted she skip the travel, move to part time, and take a semester off from her master's program. I took a breath of the dewy Hawaiian air and pushed the emotions down, refusing to give them space to fester while Jess and I were supposed to be celebrating. For the next day and a half, I tried to hide my sulking from Jessica as we drove around the island, lazed around on postcard-perfect iconic beaches, and ate snow cones. I was even cranky at the Luau.

That night, after we got back to the room from the stupid Luau (I usually love Luau's, too), Sierra called again. I was perplexed. What had happened now?! I almost sent her call to voicemail, not wanting to deal with more frustration that night. I sighed and decided to be an adult and answered the phone. Sierra screamed into my ear, "I'm going to Redmond! Redding said I was physically ready and..." She went off and I was completely lost. "What?! Hold on, slow down, how is that possible?"

Sierra slowed down her excitement and re-explained that Redding reached out to another smokejumper base, Redmond, that was set to start their rookie training next week, in two days. Since Sierra was physically fit enough to pass through Redding's first two weeks, Redmond offered her another shot. Apparently, finding fit enough humans who also have wildland fire experience is a rare commodity! Good thing, too. The caveat—Sierra would have to start the following week, back at the beginning of rookie training, in week one. This time, she would be training on the round parachutes, the chutes that she was supposed to train on in the first place before Redding had shipped her and the other rookies off to Boise.

Sierra had accepted and was driving up to Redmond, Oregon as we spoke. I couldn't believe it. Boise washed her on technique errors, and a day later, Redmond picked her up on the premise that she was physically fit and could learn how to jump on the round parachutes, which were less technical. Redmond was betting that Sierra's physical aptitude and strong resume were worth salvaging. She was given another chance. This time, I was completely dumbfounded.

Now I had to wait another five or six weeks to see if she made it through, and Sierra had to undergo an additional bout of rookie training. I hoped that her body would hold up. When constructing her training and taper, I had aimed her peak for week three, hoping that she would feel powerful through week five. If she had to go six weeks, I thought she might be able to make it. Now that she had doubled down and was in for another five or six weeks on top of the three that she'd already put in, I was extremely concerned. Nine weeks of rookie training is unheard of.

Like Groundhog Day, I wished her luck and off she went. This time to Redmond. I had less of an idea how they tested and trained rookies there. I had researched how to prepare Sierra based on Redding standards and rumors. Redmond was a US Forest Service base, same as Redding, so I figured we were close enough with our preparation strategy. However, Redmond felt like a crapshoot. The odds were heavily stacked against her. I wondered how she would feel after the six-hour drive from Boise, Idaho to Redmond, Oregon. She was physically beat up from two weeks of rookie training in Redding and one week in Boise. I wondered what her inner dialogue sounded like. Was she positive or negative? What did she think about washing out? Was she concerned about how her new rookie brothers and sisters would feel once they learned that she had just washed out at Boise? Furthermore, Sierra might end up physically falling apart. Having to endure a second "hell" week is about as rough as it gets. She had no time no rest between ending one program and starting up the next, taking just a single weekend off. After three weeks of grueling physical and mental challenges, and the psychological hit of washing out at Boise, I hoped that she was mentally strong enough to keep her wits about her. She also now had to integrate into a new group of rookies at Redmond. Hopefully they would accept her.

Over the next month, while waiting for something I could not control, I stuck to my classic style of burying myself in any work I could find. I carefully programmed for my personal clients and wrote thank you cards for our wedding guests. I worked on bolstering my database of YouTube exercise demo videos to use as hyperlinks in my online training. Jess and I exercised and went on beach walks, and in the evenings, I drank whiskey on the porch with Snowflake. At the end of each week, I'd text Sierra and check on her. She had made it through the first week at Redmond. Again, she said it was extremely tough, and again, that she had barely made it. A week went by. She was running on fumes. Another week passed, and Sierra was still going. I anxiously waited, knowing that week three was the introduction to jump protocols for the round parachutes. This was the week that she had washed at Boise, during the technical parachute training. At the end of the week, after making mistakes and learning despite the physical fatigue, she was still in. The fourth week was also tough and technically demanding, and she survived. Only one or two more weeks to go.

After almost two full months of smokejumper rookie training, Sierra called me up mid-week. When I answered, I knew immediately what had happened. Across three different bases in three different states, after training diligently and sporadically for five months, while working full-time through many sleepless nights at the San Diego fire station, while completing her second master's degree, and overcoming the death of a friend and a family member, at the age of 39 years old, Sierra passed rookie training. I really couldn't believe it. Her tone was upbeat and weathered. She mentioned how happy she was, and how the rest of her rookie crew was going to celebrate that night despite their exhaustion. Beaming, I congratulated her. I am convinced that Sierra's amazing endurance ability which she had cultivated throughout her entire life is what enabled her to press on without physical setback, and perhaps our preparatory training helped a little, too. That night, I don't know how Sierra celebrated with her fellow rookie bros, but I imagine it involved toasting and laughter and falling asleep early.

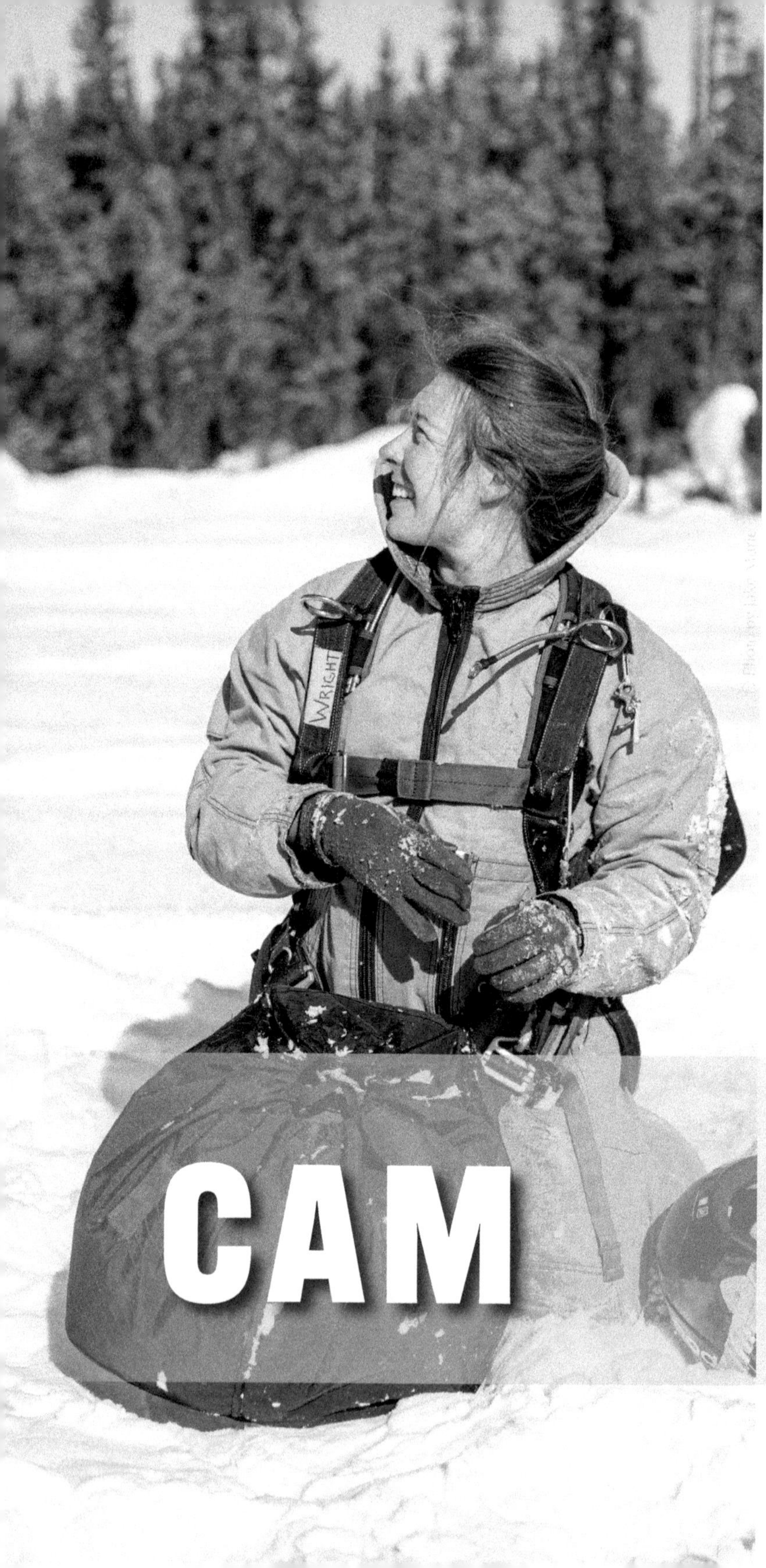

4 CAM

FOLLOWING SIERRA'S SUCCESS, MY CONFIDENCE WITH COACHING SMOKEJUMPERS INCREASED. Heidi wasn't a fluke! And neither was Sierra. Or so it seemed at that moment as I surfed on the emotional coattails of their successes. Yes, I might have lucked out drawing two talented, stubborn, and dedicated females to work with me. But we also had a lot of things right. Both athletes had arrived at rookie training pain-free and fresh. Heidi's numbers and pack test were heavily improved from the year before. I had a phone call with one of the supervisors at Boise who knew Heidi, Matt Bowers, and he said, "Heidi crushed it her third year. The previous season, she got washed on day one for failing the pack test. The next year, on the heavy pack test, she beat every male except for one guy, who was 6'2" and 200 pounds—almost ten years younger!" Heidi had built the physical fortitude to keep her mind right while learning the jump commands, enabling her to graduate. Sierra's PT strength endurance and rucking had come a long way from where she had started, and she was able to survive during eight straight weeks of smokejumper rookie training at 39 years of age. Both women had experienced exceptional physical, mental, and psychological growth over a short period of time.

After the excitement fizzled from my wedding, honeymoon, and Sierra's unusual success, I was left feeling hollow. Sure, I was proud of Sierra and myself, but I still felt flat. Floundering. The feeling seemed to stem from professional backsliding since leaving Redlands. Jess argued that I had reached the limits of my potential in Redlands, and it was time to build anew in San Diego. She was right, of course. However, knowing this didn't help. It was easy for her to say, "Cheer up and look at all this opportunity down here!" She had landed in this city with the job she desired.

A few months before, after a year of employment, I quit working at the athlete training center. I had given coaching kids a solid try. I enjoyed teaching them how to move, and I had learned much about myself, but there were difficulties at the business that I could not overcome. Also, I did not see a way there to progress professionally. At least the wildland firefighters were doing well. That was my lifeline—the fact that I could help professionals of this caliber. It gave me strength to press on.

For the next few months, I again began devoting time, energy, and creativity to building my personal business. Momentum began to grow. I worked in my oddly shaped office at the rear of my small San Diego house and wrote training programs for ten athletes from Redlands.

I also played games with Snowflake, whom we had recently invited to live inside our home (she accepted). We'd moved her into the house during the winter the year before because, at the time, she had seemed wet, cold, and miserable. She was not completely move-in ready, though. After a week, Jess and I had both begun to itch like crazy on our feet and ankles. Snow was flea-ridden. I thought that I knew what that word meant, but turns out I didn't. Me being a picker, scratched the shit out of my feet, ankles, and calves until they bled. Then we realized that old Snow had infected us with her parasites. Yuck.

We bathed her immediately, and then continued the tortuous yet loving process once a month for a while until all the fleas were gone. Since she was a white cat, once we wet her down, we could see hundreds of little dark-colored buggers scrambling around beneath her fur as we gently held her down and doused her with water and flea shampoo in our old paint-chipped, eggshell-colored, clawfoot bathtub. She wasn't crazy about the experience and kept growling and eyeballing me with a look that said, "Bloody hell... I'll get you for this."

Jess and I scrubbed the poor gal, picking off the live and dead bugs as we worked all the way down to her skin, parting rows of fur and chasing the live ones down with a flea pick, and counting each one as we went. We lost count after 200. After the bath, it became immediately apparent that she was terrified of the hairdryer and not going to sit still for that, so to dry her, I burrito-wrapped her in a couple of towels because it was cold, and the poor cat was shivering, and Jess blasted the hair drier on a light setting until she looked dazzlingly white. Before this day, we thought she was light gray, but really, she was permanently covered in a layer of street grime. She eventually forgave us, for we continued to feed her and give her toys.

We also started to give her flea pills. At first, she would eat one mixed into her food. Then she outsmarted us, and we had to mix it into her treats. That stopped working, too, and eventually I had to use the cat burrito method, shoving the pill in her mouth as she roared, claws ripping through the towel. "I'll bloody bite your face off, you two bit..." she growled. If she bit me, it still hurt despite her lack of canines. I had some marks on my hand from her gummy little unkempt British teeth.

After leaving the athlete training center, I desired to coach general population athletes again, like my glory days in Redlands. There is a world-famous CrossFit gym in San Diego named Invictus. After coaching CrossFit in Redlands for years, I should have immediately stopped into Invictus after the move, but I had mistakenly pre-judged them as a poor fit for me and put them out of my mind. I thought I wasn't a traditional CrossFit coach and decided to test other coaching avenues. However, after the athlete training center, I realized that coaching CrossFit was more enjoyable and seemed like the best way for me to maximize my creativity and growth.

I finally dropped in for a class to experience the environment. I had a blast! I was welcomed by the coach of my class, the workout was fun, and my classmates seemed friendly. The gym was big, bright, and seemed to run well. CJ, the owner, had a positive reputation according to everyone I asked. There were many videos of him on YouTube, which I watched to get a sense of his personality before attempting to land a coaching position.

The next day after my first workout, I Googled them and found an article saying that they were hiring. What timing! I excitedly spent time updating my resume and emailed it over. The response back made me blush. I had accidentally dug up an old article from years ago. Invictus wasn't currently hiring. But, with a stroke of luck, a few days later, I received another email saying they were looking to hire. The manager wrote, "I think we just sent out an ad for a part-time coach yesterday! Your timing couldn't be better." I could easily fit in coaching a few Invictus classes each week with my programming duties. After a week's time and a few interviews with coaches, managers, and CJ, I was offered a part-time position and accepted the role. The place seemed like a great fit.

I made strides with my business during the six months off between the athlete training center and Invictus. I re-learned the lesson that in-person coaching allowed me to thrive professionally. Iron sharpens iron, as the saying goes. I found the other coaches passionate, intelligent, and highly skilled, which provided me the best professional learning environment I could ask for.

It was now October 2019. I had been working at Invictus for three months. The wildfire season was coming to an end. After Sierra made it through rookie training, just like after Heidi, other female wildland firefighters began to seek me out. I chatted on the phone with a few, but none seemed serious. The leads came from Heidi, who had always been great at networking for my services. I don't know how to advertise to this specific population of athletes. Fortunate for me, Heidi did this for me by simply spreading the word to those who were interested. She told them her story, and that I had successfully trained her and another female to pass smokejumper rookie training. She told them that my system worked.

Heidi set me up with a potential smokejumper candidate, another woman. Heidi said she had a few years of wildland fire experience on an engine crew and as a hotshot. I called her up to chat. She didn't sound stoic and militaristic like Heidi and Sierra. This young lady had a sweetness about her that I had not expected to find in a wildland firefighter. On the phone, she sounded wispy and whimsical, like a Southern Bell but without the accent.

From day one, she was steadfast in her desire to become a smokejumper. She was given the green light from her supervisor on the hotshot crew to train full-time this winter and spring. A great sign. Back to the full-time athlete approach. I could write whatever I wanted again! How freeing!

She gave me her best PT marks over the phone, and I was pleasantly surprised to hear that she was on the edge of being fit enough. She didn't yet have a candidate offer, but that was normal this time of year. Rookie training candidates are offered bids 3–6 months out. Over the winter, she planned to visit the Boise and Fairbanks smokejumper bases. Another good sign. She was serious. Committed. I could sense her desire. Like Heidi, she seemed quiet. But behind that wall of silence seemed to roar a passion for her work and her life. I couldn't put my finger on it, but there was just something about her that gave me confidence in her going the distance even though she was a long way out. Months, years even. I knew some male hotshots with years of experience who applied every year to smokejumper bases and came away empty-handed.

Over the next week, she picked my brain further, and I helped assure her that I could help. She trusted Heidi's referral and quickly seemed to buy into my limited wildland fire coaching experience even though we had just met. My top selling point was my perfect 2-0 record with female smokejumpers.

Our interactions were only mildly awkward, as most athlete onboarding calls are between an unacquainted man and woman. We stumbled over each other's words as we worked to understand each other's speaking cadence. She had a long pause before answering my questions. It was uncomfortable at first until I understood that she was thinking deeply before formulating her answer, and she seemed confident doing so without the use of a filler word like "um," "like," or "ahh." Silence was enough. After getting used to her unique way of communicating, the novelty became refreshing. I left each conversation feeling reassured that she was deep, patient, and thorough.

Years later, I would find out her back story. I share that with you now to fill the gaping hole in the story of who Cam is. Just know that for the first few years of our coach-athlete relationship, I knew very little about her. All of what she wrote below was new to me years later:

> *Growing up in Vermont, wildland fire wasn't something that I had really considered or even heard about until I worked on a trail maintenance crew after college in New Hampshire. I found that I really enjoyed working outside, especially the physical challenge of it all.*
>
> *One of the guys on my trail crew talked about moving out West and getting into wildland fire. For some reason, that idea really got stuck in my head. Over the following winter, I found out as much as I could about wildland fire. I called friends of friends who worked in fire and asked them about their experience. I even called a hotshot superintendent because I was able to find his number online and asked him how I could become a hotshot. I actually met him a few years ago and said thanks for the advice. He didn't remember the phone call, but he was really glad to hear that I had stuck with it. He told me to keep working on trail crews for a few more seasons and to try and work on some sort of a federal crew and get my Red Card to fill in with a fire crew. And that is pretty much what I did.*
>
> *Through some pretty wild serendipity, I made some connections with Rocky Mountain National Park and got hired on their Trail Crew in 2015. That was such a fun summer!*
>
> *The following winter, I did my best to tell everyone that I met that I wanted to be a firefighter and ended up with a job at Mesa Verde National Park on their wildland engine in 2016. Pretty much immediately my engine captain told me that I would be well-suited to*

be a hotshot, and that I would gain a lot of experience really quickly on a hotshot crew. I was really lucky to land at Mesa Verde my first season with such supportive people. I think the FMO (Fire Management Officer) told me within the first month of me working there that I should become a smokejumper. I'm sure I laughed at the time, but I think Steve is the person that planted the idea in my mind.

The next season, 2017, I got hired as a hotshot back at Rocky Mountain NP with the Alpine Hotshots. I loved a lot of things about being on the crew—seeing so much interesting fire behavior, traveling all over the country, the camaraderie. Working for the Park Service was super cool because we got to go do prescribed burns for other National Parks, from Mount Rushmore to the Grand Canyon and Saguaro National Park.

Cam's initial strength numbers were comparable to Sierra's starting marks. She had a solid distance running capacity and background, and she knew how to powerlift, which was a strong indicator for being able to train her to handle the heavy pack test and all the rucking.

After one more talk, she agreed to work with me. After our phone conversation, I smiled, pumped my fist, and immediately yelled across the house to Jess, "I have another female smokejumper hopeful!" Jess smirked. "Good job. Time for you to spend all your free time programming again. She better listen better than Sierra, or else. What's her name?" I laughed, "Cameron. She goes by Cam. I think she's gonna be good."

WEDNESDAY, OCTOBER 23, 2019 (INITIAL TESTING)

Cam was eager to get started, so I spent that weekend glued to my brown particle board desk from Target. I hoped I could help her. I had not prepared a smokejumper last season and felt rusty. It had been two years since the start of Sierra's preparation. To refresh my memory, I went back into Heidi's sheets to explore how I structured her training. I also looked over Sierra's training to gather my thoughts. It helped. Plus, I had advanced my spreadsheet knowledge. They looked cleaner and functioned better. I felt ready.

First things first—testing. Cam had been training on her own for a few weeks post-fire season and felt fresh enough, so I asked her to complete a full PT test. Her initial marks:

	BLM High Standards	***Cam's preseason scores***	***Cam's Initial Goals***
1.5-mile Run	9:30	9:46	9:00
Pull-ups	10	6	12
Push-ups	35	33	66
Sit-ups	60	60	120
Pack Test	110 lbs., 3 miles, 65 mins.	45 lbs., 3 miles, 38 mins	110 lbs., 3 miles, 55 mins

Like Heidi, Cam thought that the Bureau of Land Management bases were the most challenging to rookie out of, so she chose that route. I liked her already. Her marks were currently just within the minimum stan-dards for Boise or Alaska, but she was below the high standards. She was 4 pull-ups shy of the high standard, 2 push-ups, and on the money for the sit-ups. She was 16 seconds slow for the run. I thought that this was a decent starting point.

I asked her where she'd like to set her initial goals to work towards by April, and she didn't really know what was possible or where she should be at that time. She didn't have a reference for how many reps of each task she would need to complete to be successful at rookie training. I knew "as many as humanly possible" was the answer, so we initially decided to double everything and aim for that.

I didn't know if doubling her PRs was possible in the short time we had to prepare. To get a glimpse of Cam's potential trajectory, I referenced against Heidi's and Sierra's outcomes. Heidi's numbers were already high before we worked together, and I helped her drive them higher, but we definitely didn't double her marks. Heidi's first year improvements averaged at 39% increases across the main three tested calisthenics:

	Heidi's Previous PRs	*Heidi's Ending Scores*	*Change (%)*
1.5-mile Run	9:30	9:02	-0:28 seconds, 5% faster
Pull-ups	16	22	+6 reps, 38% increase
Push-ups	66	95	+29 reps, 44% increase
Sit-ups	100	135	35% increase
Pack Test	Failed, washed immediately	110 lbs., 3 miles, 50:37	+35 reps, 35% increase

Sierra's improvements were more impressive. She averaged a 78% gain across the PT tasks:

	Sierra's Previous PRs	*Sierra's Ending Scores*	*Change (%)*
1.5-mile Run	10:00	9:15	(-0:45 seconds, 5.6% faster)
Pull-ups	6	13	(+7 reps, 116% increase)
Push-ups	48	78	(+30 reps, 63% increase)
Sit-ups	86	135	(+49 reps, 57% increase)
Pack Test	no mark	110 lbs., 3 miles, 57 mins	Massive improvement

Sierra's 78% gain is almost 40% higher than Heidi's improvement. This makes sense when you take into context the difference in the difficulty of progressing from 6 pull-ups to 13 versus 16 to 22. It is much more challenging to improve one's performance when they are already strong.

With confidence built upon the lessons learned through coaching Heidi and Sierra, I eagerly forged forward with Cam's planning.

After a few years, San Diego finally felt like home. I was working part time about three days a week at Invictus and writing training programs at home two other days each week. I had also stopped driving to Redlands on the weekends. Jess and I were now proud San Diego Zoo membership holders and drove there to take walks a few days a week. Our zoo time together was carefree and slow. We enjoyed getting lost together in the zoo and then trying to find our way back to head home before Jess had to leave for the start of her shift at the hospital. She had also picked up a part-time job working a couple of nightshifts a week at a tiny hospital in Coronado, a short drive over the bridge to the island. When she was at work or sleeping in from her late shift, I enjoyed going on long hikes and trail runs in Mission Trails, a park near my house. While out in the wilderness, I let my mind run wild and often found myself problem solving training dilemmas for my online athletes. When solutions arose, I made mental notes, heading home at sundown. Being my number one priority athlete this season, Cam was always top of mind.

Snowflake was a happy cat. During the days, she roamed her yard, queen of the domain. Sometimes she'd get in scrappy fights with other drifter cats in the neighborhood. She was a bullish twelve-pounder with the swollen and scarred-up face of an aging boxer, large claws, no teeth, and a temper. Now that she was on flea pills, we didn't need to bathe her as often. She still stank sometimes, and into the clawfoot tub she'd go, complete with a cat-towel burrito dry off. What a weirdo. She almost never ate all her food, which we found odd given that she was living on the street for the past unknown number of years. She was living the good life. To Jess and me, she was worth the extra effort to keep her clean, fed, and parasite-free. When we called her, she'd saunter over with her pink bejeweled "Snowflake" collar gleaming in the sunlight. She'd hop up on our lap and sit for a bit, tolerating our petting and sweet talking. Eventually she'd get irritated, growl, and hop off again. We loved her.

The only major downside to living in this location became apparent. Our house was at the back of the property, right up against the alleyway. For the past year, the tire shop that existed 30 feet down the alley from our kitchen window had sold only tires and rims, but recently, we had been experiencing some atrocious bass coming from the place. It was 9 in the morning, and I was concerned the music volume and our house walls vigorously vibrating would wake the sleeping Jessica, which was not something I was interested in dealing with, so I walked over to talk to the owner, who apologized and had the customer turn it down. The tire shop now sold speakers, turns out. Big ones.

Later that evening, after returning home from a long sunset hike in Mission Trails, I sat down at my small desk with a glass of rye and began to program the macro and mesocycles of Cam's season plan. She had not yet been picked up as a rookie candidate. However, she was actively seeking. For now, we assumed a general end date of early to mid-April of next year, 2020. That left us just over five months to get her in the best shape of her life.

For the initial assessment, I looked at Cam's age, size, strengths, and availability to train:

- 28 years old, 5'5" and about 145 lbs.
- 9:45 for the 1.5-mile out the gate, 6:30/mile pace (she seemed like a strong runner)
- Experience with barbell training (squats, deadlifts, hip thrusts)
- Some CrossFit experience
- She was not going to work this offseason!

Her physical and logistical weaknesses at this stage in the program drafting process seemed manageable. She was living in Colorado with her fiancé in a cabin. There was a gym about 45 minutes away from her house (one-way), and she only wanted to commute there twice a week due to the long drive. This forced me to get creative about how to train her at home with the limited equipment that she had available.

I decided to try a similar model with Cam that had worked for Heidi and Sierra. We focused on several training modalities:

Now that I had the modalities and a 5-month timeline, it was time to create a tab within her spreadsheet that contained all of her major trackable data: running mileage, weekly training hours, heavy pack training, speed training (running), PT scores, and I added in a new section this year that I had not utilized for either Heidi or Sierra—weekly physiological tracking. To keep track of her physiological response to the training, at the end of each week, I asked her to individually score her appetite, sleep, and mood. I decided to use a scale 0–5, where 5 is highest/best. This was to become my "canary in the coal mine" and would signal if and when she began to overreach. That way I could adjust the volume for the rest of her week or the following week to allow for greater recovery and less physical stress.

In addition to adding the physiological tracking data points, I desired to track Cam's training duration each day and week more accurately. With Heidi, I had estimated her training session duration and summed up all the time each week, increasing her work time as we headed towards her volume peak and then decreasing through the taper. With Sierra, she was so unpredictable that I hadn't counted or tracked her training hours. It was too challenging. After sitting with that problem for two years, I arrived at a simple solution in my head while hiking one day. I added a cell in the top line of each training day where Cam could write in her total training time for that day, including warm-ups and cool downs. I planned to compile her total completed minutes each week and compare that to the number of hours that I had estimated her training would take. I hoped this would help me improve accuracy with Cam's training dosage each day and week as we worked towards her volume peak in March.

I wondered what Cam's strengths and weaknesses would be during the upcoming trek towards April. Taking a look back at the other women, Heidi's PT numbers had already been stellar when I started training her, and yet she demanded that we push them higher to increase her chances for success. Sierra, on the other hand, didn't have the PT numbers that Heidi had, but she had an extreme endurance background that seemed to be her saving grace.

- **Thorough warm-ups:** I implemented many of the same warm-ups that I used for Heidi and Sierra, and I made sure to go through them all beforehand to take out some of the tasks that I no longer relied upon and added in newer stuff that I was enjoying. To keep things interesting, I utilized seven different warm-up variations and ten different cooldown stretching protocols.
- **Mobility:** After the general warm-up, I wrote in mobility drills to help prep Cam's hips, ankles, thoracic spine, scapulae, and shoulders.
- **Hiking:**
  - Heavy pack training with a linear periodization
  - Medium pack training, about half the weight of the heavy pack for that week
  - Light pack training, about one quarter the weight of the heavy pack
- **Running:** Since Cam had been running regularly before coming to me, we were able to jump right into it.
- **Strength training:** Cam knew how to deadlift and perform other resisted hinging tasks, back and front squat, bench press, strict press, push press, and some Olympic Weightlifting. She was also a fan of glute training and wanted to keep her buns in good shape, so I gladly planned to sprinkle in a healthy amount of barbell glute bridges and hip thrusts.
- **Power training:** From my track and field background, power tasks are my personal favorite. Sprints, jumps, and medicine ball throws are fun and important teaching and preparatory tasks for the body and its tissues.
- **PT work (of course):** Plenty of pull-ups, push-ups, sit-ups, and their derivatives.
- **Core training:** Heidi and Sierra both experienced many different types of core-destroying fun at rookie training, so I decided to dose Cam with a high amount of as many different tasks as I could conjure up.
- **Accessory work:** To keep her joints and tissues healthy and happy, I planned to program about 15% of Cam's training volume as accessory work. These often simple and lightly loaded or bodyweight tasks have the specific purpose of ensuring that Cam's joints and tissues withstand the amount of volume that I planned to put her through.
- **The Fun Stuff:** Cam loved to skin and cross country ski, so I planned to schedule in as much of this as she wanted. The more fun the training seems to the athlete, the less it feels like training and the more it feels like living an exciting and active life. When training becomes monotonous or tedious, the mind begins to wither, and the body soon follows. I wanted to keep her training fun and fresh, and this was one sure way to help achieve that purpose.

I didn't know Cam's mindset well enough yet to locate her strengths and weaknesses. All I had was a first impression of a quiet, deep-thinking young woman who was on the cusp of being strong enough for rookie training. I was uncertain whether she had what it took to become a smokejumper, and I was intrigued to see what she was made of over the next five months.

MONDAY, OCTOBER 28-SUNDAY, DECEMBER 8, 2019 (TRAINING BLOCK ONE, 6 WEEKS)

Jess had recently put in her two weeks' notice for her second job, which was a true noc-shift (nocturnal shift)—11:00 p.m. to 7:30 a.m. There had been stretches of time over the past year where she would work almost two weeks in a row. This had been tough on us both. It made planning travel and date nights more challenging, and sometimes Jess was quicker to frustration with me, and I reciprocated. I despised the phrase, "day in and day out" and lived as if pretending it wasn't happening would keep the feeling away. The truth is that putting one's head in the sand doesn't solve much.

The only stable thing in my life seemed to be that dirty white street cat, who was now a half-time house cat. We let her out whenever she asked. Sometimes she wasn't nice about it. Let's just say that if I was lying on the couch watching a show, and Snow was stretched out on my belly as I petted her, when she had enough pets, she'd start to swoosh her tail in my face, her frustration eventually turning into a growl. That was her cue. She needed some personal time in her yard, and out she'd go. Then I'd turn off the show and get back to work on Cam's programming, ending my Netflix break.

Fartlek runs are a form of interval training. This type of running workout is traditionally unstructured, meaning the parameters for how to perform the intervals can be loose and flexible. For example, over a 2–5 mile distance, for interval parameters, I may have athletes:

- **Use time**—30 seconds run a bit faster + 60 seconds recovery pace
- **Use distances**—100 meters push pace + 300 meters easy recovery jog
- **Use unique, flexible distances**—Run fast to the next telephone pole + slow recovery jog to the following pole
- **Strides**—30 hard strides + 50 easy-paced strides (A stride is left-right, every other step. Strides are easier to count than steps)
- **And even breathing**—Run hard for 10 full breath cycles + easy run with 25 slow recovery breaths

The parameters are limited by landscape, the athlete's unique preferences and abilities, and the creativity of the coach!

Cam's first week went well, which reassured me once more that a sizeable professional challenge was capable of injecting inspiration into the flatness that I had felt just a month ago. I had more pep in my step. I enjoyed getting to know her through the spreadsheets, the same way that Heidi, Sierra, and I had developed our coach-athlete relationships. After Cam's first running workout, a 2-mile fartlek run with 400-meters pushing her pace followed by a slow 400-meter recovery jog pattern, Cam wrote, "average pace (including warm-up) was 10:21/mile. I added on an extra 1.3 miles because it was beautiful and did an extra fartlek because one got interrupted by a barking dog. Elevation gain was 1,440 ft. Feeling good after that ... We're just here for a few days, so I'm just enjoying running in these beautiful mountains!" Cam was in Alaska visiting the smokejumper base in Fairbanks. Despite being out of town, she still wanted to begin training asap, so she made it work. A less motivated athlete would have taken the vacation as rest. Not Cam. She already knew what was at stake. Time was preciously short.

Later this week, she wrote, "8:46 pace, flat terrain. My first solo run in AK, had to make a few stops cuz I thought I heard something in the bushes... actually feeling pretty good about it because I am seriously afraid of bears, even though it was kind of slow." Reading this one made me smile. Anywhere else, and I'd write the bear comment off as paranoia. But in Alaska, bears are a definite possibility.

Perhaps the most difficult part of training smokejumper hopefuls was the remote nature of our coach/athlete relationship. I could not train them in person very often, if ever. While preparing Heidi, we had worked together in person once a month. I only worked with Sierra twice. Cam lived so far away that I might never work with her in person. I might not even meet her. I had to trust her word, and through the spreadsheets, I had to learn to read her demeanor and how much to push her and when to back off.

The rest of week one went well. No nagging injuries. She followed what I wrote and provided concise and consistent feedback. Her first heavy pack training session went well, 50 pounds for 2 miles. She completed this in 29 minutes. 14:30 miles, a great pace for an initial pack session. She liked the glute training I had written her. For pull-ups, that week in Alaska she didn't have access to a pull-up bar, so she used her ice climbing picks. In one of her pull-up workouts from week one, she wrote, "worked on starting from full extension. The last 2 were tough. (Once we get settled in for the winter, we'll have a good pull up bar—for now, the ice tools are easy to hang...)" I found this creative and a sign that Cam was willing to do what it took to be successful. Some athletes might use the excuse that they don't have a pull-up bar and skip the training. Instead, she hung her ice picks over a beam in the cabin and got to work. Was this optimal? Nope. Was it pretty great? Yep, I thought so.

For her push-ups this week, I asked her to hit multiple sets of 10—12 reps. This is about 33% of her max reps. In her feedback, she had trouble completing the last few repetitions on her last set, so for next week, I decided to drop the reps to a more easily attainable target. I had learned this lesson the hard way in the past with athletes. Ask an athlete if they want to go up in reps or stay the same, almost everyone chooses to go up. However, most will benefit from keeping their repetitions per set low to keep quality high. The simple way to add volume is to increase the total number of sets. This is safe and effective. This is a principle I learned from reading Pavel Tsatsouline's PlanStrong course manual. He also bakes this concept into almost every training book he writes. Stay away from lactate most of the time. Keep quality high, and structure sets, reps, resistance, and rest periods to accomplish this.

To ensure that I coached Cam to move efficiently, I used an app called Marco Polo. It's a video chatting app. Any time she had technique or training-related questions, she sent me videos. This week, I immediately sent her a video instructing how to optimize her sit-up technique. In a video she sent me, she was sitting up too high on her sit-ups and each rep took too much time. The standard for testing was "tips of elbows touching the top of the knees." I sent her a video to teach this, and once she practiced the technique, she improved immediately. She wrote, "these felt way easier! I know I still have some work to do to get the right technique every time, but it was much easier." I love when corrections work the first time.

I felt that she trusted me to guide her, and she followed what I asked. Her feedback in the spreadsheets, texts, and through videos was exactly what I needed to confidently continue driving her forward with minimal risk. After a single week in, we were making progress. Faster sit-ups. Dialing in her other tasks. That first heavy pack training session was fast. I attributed these initial improvements to Cam's desire and consistency. Ever since she'd knocked out those pull-ups on vacation in Alaska while hanging from ice climbing axes, I knew she was different. Since then, she had charged forwards, even pushing through an acute illness. Early on, she got food poisoning mid-week and pushed through anyway, finishing her training that day and the next. This was a sign to me that she was tough and committed, even at this early stage. She could have easily skipped a few workouts to recover, but she didn't. She knew what was on the line and that every training session mattered.

Immediate progress is expected with an athlete like Cam who is rough or unpolished, still working through developmental stages. Sure, she was faster and stronger than most females on the planet, but that wouldn't get her a candidate offer. She would have to prove that she was stellar amongst the other candidates applying for the BLM smokejumper bases. Her application was competing with the males—the same as with Heidi and Sierra.

When Cam sent me her first form check Marco Polo video, I found it cute that she seemed nervous. I had spent the past few years using video coaching with my athletes, so to me, making videos was now run-of-the-mill. I had forgotten how initially weird and awkward talking to a camera could be. Cam came off as shy, which I thought was a stark juxtaposition to her athletic ability and accompanying massive physical and professional goals.

At the end of the week, she ran 8.5 miles at conversational pace and afterwards felt one of her hips talking to her, so she stretched it out and it felt better after that. In addition, while performing side planks, her left shoulder felt less stable than her right. I was hyper observant of her feedback this week. On my radar, I now had her hip and left shoulder. Neither the hip nor shoulder were injured, but they were lacking something, either mobility, stability, or both. For now, I planned to simply pay attention to them. I hoped that the training was correctly balanced to help align these asymmetries.

Cam was in Alaska for a few more weeks. I progressed her PT training and accessory work by one set (about 20% more volume) and added 10% to her running volume, bringing her up to 22 miles this week. Her feedback steadily began to show me her personality and work ethic. Midweek, she wrote, "my R hip is a little sore after today. I was a little crunched for time and rushed the warm up/ cool down. Will stretch & ice tonight, and try not to rush in the future." This was huge. Already within the second week, she noticed that her warm-up and cool down had a significant effect on how she felt. Many athletes don't learn this lesson until it's too late. It is easy when training alone without the in-person guidance of a coach to skip or shorten warm-ups and completely omit the cool down and mobility work. Cam's feedback also let me know that her right hip the week before wasn't a one-off. It was now becoming a trend and would need to be addressed directly.

Cam added a cool data stream for me to sift through. In week two, for some of her runs, she inserted a Strava link into the sheets. Strava is an online platform that allows users to link their fitness tracker data for runs, bike rides, hikes, skiing, etc. Users can add you as a friend, allowing you to follow their performances, including a map of their route and the paces of each mile. I enjoyed viewing the maps of her running and hiking routes.

Heavy pack training was just as important for Cam as it was for the previous two women. Each week for this first month, I increased her heavy pack training parameters, either load or distance:

	Pack Weight	*Distance*	*Time*	*Pace*
Week 1	50 lbs.	2 miles	29 minutes	14:30/mile
Week 2	50 lbs.	3 miles	48 minutes	16:00/mile
Week 3	60 lbs.	3 miles	55 minutes	18:20/mile
Week 4	65 lbs.	3 miles	55 minutes	18:20/mile

She took a few weeks off from heavy pack training after week four due to weather and travel. These times were a good starting point. I hoped that she would continue to maintain this sub-65-minute pace as the pack weight steadily crept upwards to 110 pounds.

For accessory work, I started her off with a variety of tasks, most of them isometric in nature during this first mesocycle. She handled the core and hip stability well. The only task she struggled with was a handstand hold on a wall. I like programming handstand holds for athletes because it is a simple and brutal shoulder stability and mobility task, and it also involves body awareness and a tucking of the "tail," or activation of the glutes and abdominals to maintain optimal posture through the pelvis, spine, and shoulders. The first week, she handled 30 seconds, and it seemed like no problem. Week two, I bumped the hold duration up to 35 seconds, and she couldn't complete this task. The third week, we backed off to 25 seconds and she crushed it but still felt it was too much. I had simply started her off at too long of a hold duration. We ended with sets of 22 second holds, and that seemed about perfect. She completed multiple rounds of this hold, building volume.

Throughout the last few weeks in Alaska, Cam made a strong effort to complete her training as it was written. She wrote, "had a bit of trouble improvising the right weight. The chunk of metal was a little too slippery to hold, so I tied two 25 lb plates together and they worked ok." I had written some weighted walking lunges for her at 40 pounds, and she didn't have an implement that weight, so she improvised. She literally used a chunk of metal as resistance for squats and lunges while staying at the cabin. How resourceful! Why buy a barbell when you have hunks of metal lying around?

Since week two, I had been testing out different mobility tasks to help Cam's right hip. I wrote in some hip CARs (a CAR is an acronym for Controlled Articular Rotations, which is a fancy way of saying "moving the joint through its full range of motion"), and she noticed a lack of range in her right hip during this task, the same side that was becoming fatigued more quickly on her long runs. I excitedly wrote back to her in the spreadsheets that I would add this task to her warm-ups three days a week from now on until we found a better drill or her hip issue cleared up. In week three, she also began to make headway here, stating, "I felt strong today! The pull/push/sit went really smoothly, and I felt like I was able to do all of the reps without struggling or losing form. The lunges were still a challenge ... but I was conscious of my hip alignment." I didn't realize that I was holding physical stress in my body about Cam's hip. When I read this, I exhaled deeply, relieved. If not nipped in the bud, this type of issue can nag for a long time.

> Cam knew her hip issue was sapping her of efficiency and needed to be addressed. However, sometimes athletes think that an issue as "small" as an irritated hip only causes localized pain. From what I have seen, any issue, especially hip pain, causes inefficiencies above that joint (spine-neck-shoulder) and below, too (knee-ankle-foot). When explaining this, I ask my athletes to imagine a robot with a metal skeleton and plastic joints. If that robot has one hip joint that has poor range of motion for whatever reason, how does that affect the rest of the robot's function? The hip issue actually causes the foot to strike the ground differently, and over thousands of steps running and hiking across weeks and months, if not addressed, can cause major damage.

Each week, I wrote a "fun day" for Wednesdays. I suggested that Cam could do yoga, rock climbing, skiing, or something else active and enjoyable to break the potential monotony of training for six months straight. This tactic worked well for Heidi, and Sierra naturally did this by going off-script often and taking multiple vacations during her training. In week four, it had snowed enough the weekend before, so Cam began her ski season with a 1.5-hour Nordic session. This fired me up! I could tell from her feedback that she was excited and happy. These small and meaningful experiences are powerful in keeping the athlete's morale high as they push 5–6 days a week for months on end. I knew that we were only one month in, but it felt like we were finding a rhythm. It felt like a locomotive starting up. Slow, steady, building momentum. I could feel the power behind her work ethic and motivation. No, it was deeper than motivation. Motivation is fleeting. If we all waited until we were motivated to do the things that mattered, nothing would get done. Cam was headed towards an obsession with preparing for smokejumper rookie training.

MONDAY, DECEMBER 9, 2019-SUNDAY, JANUARY 26, 2020 (TRAINING BLOCK TWO, 7 WEEKS)

My sleep schedule was still a mess. I wasn't working out nearly enough, and that was taking a heavy toll on my mindset and motivation. It was also a busy day at the tire shop, and my house was shaking. After walking out and asking them to turn it down, I walked back in to see Jess was awake and smiling like a kid who had stolen a ring pop from a gas station. It was now December, Jessica's favorite month. I couldn't help but perking up a bit due to my wife who was exuding happiness. Jess gleefully demanded that we buy a real Christmas tree from Home Depot and decorate it, along with stocking the house full of Santa dolls on shelves, wreaths, and hanging Christmas lights on everything. Growing up, my family used the same plastic Christmas tree for my whole childhood. I had always assumed that real trees were too messy. After years of experience with real trees, I was right. However, Jess demanded it.

We took that Saturday afternoon and selected our perfect little Douglas fir 7-footer, dragged it into our tiny house, and spent the evening decorating while Jess played Christmas music way too loud. We packed the tree tightly full of lights, ornaments, garland, streams of red and white fabric, all topped with a large and creepy Santa head instead of a star. Snowflake watched wearily from the far corner of the room. The tree looked overstuffed if you asked me. Jess thought we needed more decorations on the damn tree. Her Christmas decorating spirit has always been much greater than mine. I found it funny and cute to watch her get all wiggly-excited about Christmas, presents, decorating, and baking. Her spirit cheered me up. I began to look forward to the upcoming season of licking the batter off the baking utensils for her. She does have a natural baking ability, and I was about to reap the benefits for the next month. As I programmed, I'd snack on Jess's sugar cookies and Russian tea cakes. The sugar helped perk me up as well, momentarily stoking my creativity.

In Cam's largest volume week of training block one, she had peaked her training at 10 hours and just over 29 miles covered through hiking and running. Her body had seemed to hold up because her right hip and left shoulder improved, and no new issues arose.

In this second training block, my focus for Cam was to build volume with running, hiking, and PT while working to improve her strength, mobility, and stability imbalances. She was now living back in Colorado, and ski season was approaching.

During the first week of this new block, Cam's right quadricep began to act up. Yes, the quad on the same side as her hip issue. I cut her sprinting the following week and upped the posterior chain training, adding in more hinging and glute training tasks. It seemed like Cam was quad-dominant, a term used to describe an athlete whose body has learned to solve physical situations using the musculature of the front of the legs more so than the back. She often chose to squat in situations that behoove hinging. This is often accompanied by weakness in the hamstrings and glutes, so I hoped that increasing the strength of those tissues would help balance out her hip and leg strength.

Oddly enough, Cam's push-up endurance began to decrease each week. Usually, some form of improvement is noticeable on a weekly basis through working sets feeling easier or a decrease in soreness after training at a similar volume to the previous week. I didn't see either of those improvements, so instead of pushing further, in the middle of this block, I decreased volume to allow her body to adjust.

Three weeks into the block, Cam began to ski regularly. I again wrote in for her to make Wednesday a "fun" day. After a Wednesday on the slopes, she wrote, "full day of skiing! Wasn't a ton of cardio, but my legs were tired at the end of the day. I skied for 6 hours today (if that counts ...)"

At the end of this, she was asking me how much of her time skiing we could attribute to her weekly training hour log. I assumed about half, and we used that ratio for the rest of the season.

Conversations like this occurred through the spreadsheets. In fact, Cam and I communicated almost exclusively through the spreadsheet (daily), and text messages on Mondays and Fridays. Rarely did she send me form check videos through Marco Polo. And we didn't speak on the phone too often. While this may sound like a suboptimal way to communicate in a coach-athlete relationship, especially when coaching an athlete through a dense and complicated program, in my experience, these communication channels are sound enough for me to learn everything that I need to know about an athlete using a few simple touchpoints. I have been able to glean an athlete's strengths, limitations, unique abilities, recovery speed for different body parts and systems, mindset, and of course, their personality.

Sometimes, instead of hiking or running, Cam completed a different physical challenge. She wrote, "I can't get my watch to upload, but I probably hiked for about 90 minutes. I walked for 2 miles with my ice gear, then skinned to the ski hill, did a few hot laps skinning up, then skied up an unplowed road for about 45 minutes. I wasn't carrying 25 pounds while skiing, but I did have my pow skis on, so I feel like it was more strenuous than carrying 25 lbs. fun day!"

After reading this, I realized that Cam's idea of fun was in direct alignment with her training goals. This type of activity is incredibly challenging, both mentally and physically, and takes a long time. I thought this was exactly what she needed, and it served a dual purpose—fun.

Cam didn't have a smokejumper candidate bid, yet. If she was concerned about this, she kept it to herself. Since Cam was in the off-season between her in-season job on a hotshot crew, she was simply giving up leisure time to train for hours each day. Some wildland firefighters work year-round on base, but many take the off-season to travel, ski, and rest. If she didn't get a bid to smokejump this year, Cam could return to her hotshot crew for another season. It wouldn't be the end of the world for her, but she was dedicating herself completely to the journey, and not being given an opportunity to test herself would be frustrating for us both.

Cam was interested in jumping at a BLM base. Her top choices were Boise and Fairbanks. In the middle of this training block, Boise called and asked her to complete a timed 1.5-mile run. She went out the next Monday morning and completed the run in less than 10 minutes, at 6:37/mile pace. She thought it could have been faster, but I was happy with that time at this stage in her training, especially given the cold weather, snow, and mud. Testing conditions were not ideal.

There were some training conflicts with Cam's extra physical activities. She wrote, "I also ice climbed (I thought fairly moderately) but I was pretty tired in the gym. I will try my best to go to the gym before ice climbing in the future! Total climbing time this morning was probably 1 hour, plus half hour of hiking, and a little skiing (can't seem to help myself when the getting is good!)"

Her pull-up max the week before this was 7 reps (almost 8, she wrote!) but this week after ice climbing, she could only squeeze out 5 reps. This clearly illustrates the taxing nature of her ice climbing and skiing. It must have a meaningful training effect, I thought to myself, but it was difficult to quantify the training volume. How can you compare ice climbing for a certain amount of time to doing a total of X number of pull-ups? Too hard to tell. On a better note, on this same training day, her sit-ups went really well. Her technique and speed were coming along beautifully. Later this week, Cam wrote into the spreadsheets that her left shoulder began to catch up with the strength of her right. I breathed a sigh of relief. It's a good sign when most of an athlete's training session goes to plan, even if the pull-ups were off.

There is no tone in the spreadsheets or text messages, so I must guess. I use my intuition, and the relationship relies on a massive amount of trust. I trusted that Cam was being honest with me and not leaving anything out of her feedback. If she told me that everything felt fine one week even though her foot hurt, that was a sign to me that I could push her a little further the next week because, from my end, everything was fine. If she was holding back pertinent feedback like a nagging foot issue and I pushed her, and her foot got worse, then we'd be in a predicament. I didn't have to tell Cam to be honest with me. The fact that she was busting her ass in training and paying me to help her attain very clear goals was enough for me. I had complete faith that she was telling me all that I needed to know to help her. I also trusted the structure of our training and feedback channels acting as sieves to catch any physical, mental, or emotional issues that might arise. I also felt that Cam trusted me to provide her all that she needed and nothing she didn't. I always attempt to create this with my athletes. It was quite an experience remotely coaching Cam with this level of complexity and the enormity of her goals.

This was the sweet spot in the training journey. Things had really just begun. Cam's progress was noticeably upwards each week, and her body was responding beautifully. When things are going well with my athletes, especially with athletes like Cam when I am heavily emotionally invested, life's other trials and tribulations seem minuscule and I feel powerful. I live with a glean in my eye and have a wink at the ready. I had been coaching for a decade at this point and knew this superhuman feeling was bound to end any day, though. As training volume increased towards the necessary amounts that Cam would need to endure, we would begin to expose weaknesses, cracks in her seemingly unbreakable body and mind. I hoped that I had the skill to help her through when that time came.

Post-training foot care and lower leg maintenance is essential to athletes who put in many physical miles on their body. If an athlete's body is conditioned to cover 30 training miles in a week and progress over the next few months to 50 miles, all the structures and tissues of their body must adapt to handle the extra stress. Bone becomes denser, connective tissues thicker, fascia aligns to support the most persistent patterns of movement, muscle becomes more efficient. As these tissues adapt to the demands placed upon them, the athlete must ensure they are caring for their tissues and joints. I have found the best way to care for tissues and joints is to keep them pliable, mobile, and stable by incorporating post-training care of the lower legs:

- Pliability
  - Foam roll calves, shins
  - PVC, golf ball, or lacrosse ball roll the arches of the feet
- Stability
  - "Weird walks" on balls of feet, on the heels, on the inner and outer foot arches
  - Calf raises and shin strengthening through ankle dorsiflexion tasks
- Mobility
  - Completing stability tasks through full ranges of motion
  - Ankle and hip CARs. If the hips aren't moving well, that changes function at the foot and vice versa

All throughout the first 10 weeks of training, Cam's appetite, sleep, and recovery feedback were 4s and 5s out of 5. I loved that. It suggested to me that everything was going to plan. The only questionable pieces were her right quad and now her shins. They began to speak up the week before. I had learned how to address shin splints at U of I. It's common in track and field for athletes to develop foot and lower leg issues like this. Once the issue shows up, if you don't act immediately, it can progress to a point where training and competitions are severely affected. I decreased her sprint training and suggested that she double down on post-training foot care and lower leg maintenance. Even though we had a plan, I was concerned. Shin splints, even the hint of them, is never a good sign. It signifies the balance between stress and recovery is off. We didn't have time to back off.

Cam's total average weekly training time for this second block increased from 8.8 hours/week to 12.2 hours/week due to all her ice climbing, backcountry skiing, Nordic skiing, and skate skiing. She just loved getting out in the elements and challenging herself. I thought her extra training was worthwhile as long as she completed her preparatory work. If she was accepted for rookie training and showed up with a massive work capacity built up from various skiing types and ice climbing, even though her legs, heart, and lungs might be able to last, she most likely wouldn't make it through due to the sheer volume of PT. She wasn't ready, yet. Good thing we still had three months left to train.

Even though I was excited about the direction of her training, for Cam who was in the trenches grinding 6 days a week, it could be mentally tough and lonely. In week 11, on a Tuesday, Cam skipped a training day. She wrote, "I did not do it this week. I got super bummed because I thought I didn't get an interview with either base, and motivation was really low. But I do have interviews with both bases next Tuesday! It won't happen again. And I got a pull up bar at home." Even though she had a tough day, this was good news. Now she could train pull-ups at home without having to travel to the gym or perform them on her ice picks! I did not tell her, but I was also concerned that she didn't yet have a candidate offer.

In the second week of January during week 12 of her training, she completed her first official PT test for the Boise and Fairbanks bases:

	BLM High Standards	*Initial Goals*	*Late October Marks*	*Mid-January Marks*
1.5-mile Run	9:30	9:00	9:46	9:42 (4-second PR)
Pull-ups	10	12	6	8 (tied PR)
Push-ups	35	66	33	36 (3-rep PR)
Sit-ups	60	120	60	104 (44-rep PR)
Pack Test	110 lbs., 3 miles, 65 mins	110 lbs., 3 miles, 55 mins	45 lbs., 3 miles, 38 mins	80 lbs., 3 miles, 58 mins

I was very pleased with these outcomes. Cam wanted more, and I assured her that she would get faster once we began training for speed. With her nagging quad and now her shins, and the snowy and muddy terrain, it was difficult to run fast. I wanted to heal her up before focusing on increasing running speed through sprints, intervals, and repeats. I feared that introducing this type of training too early would worsen her current issues. Plus, good luck running fast in the mud and snow.

A few days later, her back began to hurt. I was beginning to elevate my level of concern. I assumed this was caused by the same underlying issue as her quad—a weak posterior chain and that poor right hip. All the training volume didn't help, either. If her hips were uneven or out of position, continuing to pile on training volume would be problematic. If we had more time, she could rest for a week or two and then we could build back up slowly with an emphasis on improving her posture. We didn't have that luxury. Her next PT test check-in was three weeks out, and then every other week after that until the start of rookie training. We had to find a way to heal her while she continued to train. This is not ideal. Risky business.

MONDAY, JANUARY 27-SUNDAY, MARCH 8, 2020 (TRAINING BLOCK THREE, 6 WEEKS)

For Christmas, Jess bought me a book called *Natural Born Heroes*, and it was firing up my motivation to get out into nature and run. I had improved my diet within the past two weeks, and the energy from that change was compounding with my excitement from the book, and now I was waking up earlier, full of energy, training more frequently, and enjoying my coaching at Invictus even more. I had accepted a full-time position the month before. My excitement for being alive was fueling my creativity for Cam's programming. It had been a while since I had felt like this. Life felt full of promise and excitement. Cam was a great challenge. Invictus was, too, and provided rich professional soil for me to set deep roots. After two and a half years in San Diego, it was finally beginning to feel like home.

Now that Snowflake was living with us full time, she made herself comfortable on my lap while I sat at my desk in the back office. While programming, I would gently pet Snow. Eventually, she'd begin to get annoyed with me, growl, and then jump down to go do whatever cats do, leaving me to my work.

In Cam's spreadsheets, I began to label each week with the number of weeks left until our hypothetical rookie training date. We were just 12 weeks out! She still had not landed a smokejumper candidate offer. We continued to train as if she had. I began to program more specific training, asking Cam to stop in the middle of a hike or a run and perform exercises. Cam wrote, "How do I get myself to like doing burpees in the snow?" I wrote back, "Pretend you are a baby polar bear."

In this third training block, I progressed Cam's volumes and intensities further. Her heavy pack training was now at 90—100 pounds. She was covering 30—40 weekly miles of running, hiking, and skate-skiing. I had planned for her average training hours each week to hover around 14—16, but outside of her gym training, she spent a ton of extra hours skiing. This pushed her average weekly training hours up to 15.5, and three of her heaviest volume training weeks were beyond 19 hours.

She completed three PT tests during this block, one every other week. As I have discussed before, I am not a fan of frequent testing because each testing session takes away from a day of training. Compared to training, testing is more taxing, both physically and mentally. However, I understand the rookie trainers thought Cam was on the borderline with her physical capacities, so they checked in frequently to see if she was moving in the right direction.

Here were her PT scores:

	PT Test 4	*PT Test 5*	*PT Test 6*
Date	2/3/2020	2/17/2020	3/3/2020
Location	Colorado	Colorado	Colorado
Pull-ups	10	10	10
Push-ups	37	37	39
Sit-ups	97	75	85
1.5 Mile Run	9:45	9:40	9:21

The highlighted scores are personal bests. Cam was concerned that her pull-ups and push-ups were not improving. I felt differently. I knew that she was consistently scoring beyond the minimum standards, which was all she needed, for now. Throughout these weeks, I placed more value on building volume than I did on maximizing her performance on the PT tests. If Cam arrived at rookie training and had a strong PT score, but we didn't train enough volume beforehand, she wouldn't last a week. I was pleased that her run was improving despite the lack of speed work. We had just recently begun to implement some faster fartlek training, but up until this point, all her endurance training was slow volume building, and much of that was skiing. Skiing is great for the legs and cardiovascular system, but it's not going to improve running speed, that's certain. The outdoor conditions in Colorado in February and early March were still snowy, cold, and muddy. Fast running was tough in the mud, and I couldn't ask her to rest between intervals for too long due to the low temperatures, so we relied on 30–60 second intervals of work and rest to push her speed.

About this time, mindset became important to Cam. Cultivating mental fortitude had proven valuable to Heidi, but you can't force an athlete to it. They must believe for it to work. If Cam only went through the motions with mental training, it would be a waste of time. However, after months of training, she finally took it up on her own and began to fill in her feedback for mindset training. I thought this was a wonderful addition to her preparation. She was realizing that her mindset would play a critical role.

Even though Cam's training weeks were becoming very long, 3–4 hours of daily training for 6 days a week, her weekly average ratings for mood, appetite, and sleep were still in the 4–5 out of 5 range, which let me know that she was recovering well. This made me smile, followed by a chuckle. She was undergoing some serious training volume and keeping a cool head. She seemed to be a great smokejumper candidate. I just hoped that a base would pick her up.

MONDAY, MARCH 9-22, 2020 (TRAINING BLOCK FOUR, THE PEAK WEEKS, 2 WEEKS)

After almost five months of hard work through consistent training, Boise placed her as an alternate, meaning if one of the other rookie candidates could not attend, then she would step into their spot. It was better than nothing. Cam's lack of a full candidate offer was disconcerting. This weighed on me. Cam must have felt immense pressure to earn a full position at Boise or Fairbanks. She had put everything on the line. She had thrown all of herself into the preparation process. She did not work. She trained full time. She had not taken time off in the off-season after her last wildland fire season. She had only taken one trip to Alaska, and that was to visit the smokejumper base in Fairbanks, and she had trained throughout that entire trip. Not much of a vacation.

As focused as I was with Cam, I was also training a dozen other athletes, including Heidi (for the third year in a row). Heidi's goal this year was similar to last year: crush the Boise Smokejumper PT test at the beginning of the wildland fire season, which was fast approaching. My wildland fire coaching was expanding. Heidi's boyfriend was also a wildland firefighter, and he was having some issues with jumper's knee, so I had helped him fix his imbalances during the past few months. He was a beast. I was also coaching a female helitack firefighter who had also been recruited by Heidi to work with me. Heidi was my wildland fire agent.

The full-time coaching at Invictus was becoming more manageable. The first few months of full-time coaching were a good stress. I soaked up how other coaches solved problems. How did they phrase their coaching cues? What new effective tasks from their warm-ups could I use with my athletes? Who were they following for continuing education? And perhaps most useful, when I had questions about physical issues with my online athletes, I could rely on asking CJ and the other coaches how they would approach the situation. I was forming a solid professional network.

At the end of the previous training cycle, for the last two weeks I deloaded Cam to prepare her for the training that was to come. The next two weeks comprised the peak of Cam's training. In week 20, she covered 44.1 miles in total across her running, hiking, ice climbing, and skiing. The next week, she pushed to 45.8 miles! This is very high training volume for a smokejumper. However, the amount was specific to her. With all the skiing and cold, muddy conditions in Colorado, time spent moving was all we could do for many months. This added up to a ton of miles and hours. While this isn't great for speed development, it's excellent for preparing the body and mind for undergoing and recovering from large chunks of daily physical exertion. Cam's physiological data held up during this time, suggesting that her body was recovering well. Yes, her PT numbers were stagnating, which is a sign that her recovery ability was close to maxed out, but I was still willing to sacrifice the rate of her PRs to pile more wood on the training volume bonfire. I believed that total training volume was more important to Cam's success at rookie training than a large PT score. While impressive, a high score does not get one through rookie training. It might only get you through day one.

In addition to the running and hiking, Cam's PT training totaled 130 pull-ups, more than 300 push-ups, and 600 sit-ups in week 21. I wrote each aspect of this training into her weekdays, leaving Saturday and Sunday as rest days for her to recover. This pushed her training to 5 hours each day. She was almost ready, and time was drawing near.

During her volume peak week, she completed one final PT test, marking 10 pull-ups (tied her PR), 41 push-ups (a new PR), 77 sit-ups (much lower than her PR), and 9:55 in the 1.5-mile run. She ran a new route with more hills than she expected, which slowed her down. I was once again pleased with this test. It showed me that Cam was still heavily fatigued, which was expected after all the training hours, reps, and miles. And yet she still held strong with her pull-ups and improved slightly in her push-ups. I think she scored low in her sit-ups because I had programmed over 1,000 reps during those two weeks, and her core was toast.

Cam also crushed the heavy pack, now at 110 pounds. She completed the 3 x 1 mile training with rest between each mile in 60 minutes, and the next week, 2 straight miles in 40 minutes. It looked like she would just sneak in under the 65-minute time cap.

For specific training, one day I had Cam complete a long ruck. She wrote, "my garmin app says it was 4,200 ft gain, in the rain and snow. telling myself: GET TOUGH, carrying 40 lbs." This hike was 9 miles and took her 4 hours. I loved reading this. And I got to learn Cam's personal mantra! I don't ask my athletes for this type of information and enjoy letting them own part of their process. I love this strategy of layering in a training mantra during the toughest sessions. After hundreds of successful experiences utilizing a specific mantra, the power of what we say to ourselves compounds and can have a massively powerful effect on how we respond to stressful situations. I imagine that practicing a mantra over many years has measurable effects on neurochemicals, hormones, and metabolism, which all play critical roles in buttressing athletes when they need it most.

Near the end of this crazy week, I wrote her a large chunk of pull-ups, push-ups, and sit-ups with the option of breaking up the total reps of each task as she saw fit. She decided to do an unbroken and large set to begin her chunk of pull-ups and pushed her max up to 11 reps! I laughed, sparking Jess to ask what was so funny. She had just woken up and was making coffee. "Cam, 11 pull-ups!" I said. Jess responded, "Wow, on her peak week?" I laughed again, happy to realize that Jess knew how tough it was to improve at this time.

To add her final stamp on this hellacious training week, instead of resting Saturday, Cam completed an 8-mile run in a little over an hour, followed by a 4-hour bike ride. Her endurance capacity was ready. I hoped it would be enough.

MONDAY, MARCH 23-SUNDAY, APRIL 19, 2020 (THE FINAL TAPER, 4 WEEKS)

I felt that Cam could use a longer and steadier taper than Heidi and Sierra. I'm not sure why I felt that way, but it seemed to fit. Call it intuition. Her physical capacities were just beyond what she needed. She had worked diligently over the past five months. She already handled 110-pound heavy pack, and she was within the time cap. Her PT scores were now beyond the high standards, and she was implementing mental training drills a few days a week in addition to her 4-hour gritty ruck session with exercises, and 8-hour backcountry ski excursions.

With two weeks left before the possible start of rookie training at Boise, Cam completed her final PT test and sent in her data. She wrote in her marks. "11 pull (so close to 12!), 52 push, 99 sit, 9:45 1.5 mi on a track—feeling a little disappointed I wasn't faster today ..." Like most athletes, she focused on the one area that didn't improve. Within a single week of tapering, her pull-ups had already jumped almost two reps, her push-ups up 11 reps, and her sit-ups were back up, close to 100. Yes, the run could have been faster, but I knew that she would run her fastest at rookie training after the completion of the full taper, if they gave her the chance. In another two weeks of tapering, I imagined that Cam would gain another pull-up or two, another 10 push-ups, and a bunch of sit-ups. I had also planned for her to perform some higher quality speed work as the weather and ground conditions became friendlier.

Physically, it seemed that Cam was right on the edge of prepared. Her PT scores were decent, but not great. Her hiking and running were strong. She handled the heavy pack well and seemed to have the endurance to train all day long. Her mindset had progressed well throughout our training, too. I badly wanted her to get a shot this season, but deep down I knew the smokejumper bases may not want to take a risk on her. Hiring a smokejumper who was right on the edge of physically ready was risky. Recruiting time is precious, and rookie training itself, potentially dangerous.

At the end of that week, I received a rare phone call from Cam. When I answered, I knew something was wrong. I could tell she was upset. Then she hit me with the news. She got word from Boise. The window had closed. All the rookie training candidates had shown up, and they did not need any alternates this year. Her smokejumper journey was over this season. I congratulated her for making it this far. I told her how proud I was of her effort and growth. With a palpable sadness in her voice, she thanked me for my help.

After hanging up, I felt deflated. All that programming work in the back office trying to ignore the bass from the tire shop while Snowflake sat on my desk trying her best to type me coded messages, gone, with nothing to show for it but a single shared epic spreadsheet. I told Jess, and she gave me a tight hug and asked, "What happens now?" I wasn't sure. Wait and see, I guess.

During the next week, my mind wandered to Cam, how hard she had worked, and how she had missed her shot this year. Retrospectively, the more I thought about the situation, the more I began to see this as a blessing in disguise. She had come a long way over the past five months of training, that was for sure, but I didn't think she had a strong chance of making it through rookie training this year. She would have to wait until next season. During the summer of 2020, Cam worked on Durango Helitack. It was the start of Covid, and she had to be apart from her boyfriend, Andy, for 6 months. He lived and worked in Alaska on a fishing boat. It was brutal for her.

When smokejumper bases recruit candidates for rookie training, they spend time and money selecting wildland firefighters who they think will make a good fit. They genuinely want each candidate to show up physically and mentally prepared. They would love for every candidate to make it through rookie training. However, somewhere between 25 - 50% of smokejumper candidates fail to complete rookie training due to injury, illness, or washing out from physical inadequacy or technical reasons. I think Boise and Fairbanks must have thought that Cam wasn't physically ready this year, or maybe they had enough candidates and hoped that she would apply again next season. Time would tell.

The middle of 2020 was a blur for me, and the world, it seemed. Masks, fear, and uncertainty swept through society. Covid 19 had shut the world down. At home, Jess and I did our best to keep each other entertained. We spent hours each week walking around our neighborhood or taking a short drive to Coronado Island to walk on the beach. We were fortunate to have the garage gym, which went a long way in helping us keep our sanity through what seemed like madness. One thing was certain. The tire shop was still selling subwoofers, and business was booming.

I continued to write training plans for my athletes and added a Zoom training feature for anyone interested. The doors were shut at Invictus for 88 straight days, and during that time, they provided us coaches about twenty hours a week of Zoom coaching and member retention work to build morale in our community and keep us employed. Everyone got to know Snowflake well. She was featured in a few of my YouTube movement instructional videos and loved sitting on my lap when I coached virtually. She constantly walked across my keyboard, once managing to change the settings, and I still haven't figured out how to fix them. The volume control is forever broken. For Jess, work didn't change much except they were doing hundreds of Covid tests in the lab each day. She still worked full time, but business slowed down considerably due to the reduction of elected procedures.

The only trip Jess and I took together that summer was to Las Vegas for the 4th of July. There wasn't much open, and the indoor mask mandate was in place, so instead of following our usual MO (pool parties, clubs, and craps), we sat in our hotel room with a few friends and through our window watched the fireworks explode all over the valley from 250 feet up. It was a serene experience, all that soundless color. I counted twenty firework explosions every 10 seconds. Then I caught myself counting. Of course, I would be mathing "fireworks per minute." It's hard to shut my brain off. We sipped our drinks and watched the explosions for an hour before falling asleep.

At the end of the summer, on a whim, one of my friends randomly invited me to go whitewater rafting with him on the American River in Northern California. I had tagged along on the same trip with him and his wife a few years before, and it was exhilarating. After being cooped up in the house all year, I craved adrenaline! It was exactly what I needed. I felt replenished and ready to conquer the world. My programming clients always benefit when I'm living with inspiration. I had recently checked in on Cam, and it looked like she was planning to start back up with programming again for the 2021 smokejumper season. She'd be home in late October. I was ready.

CAM 2.0

The summer came and went, and now we were deep into the fall. November 2020 was mentally the most challenging of my life. I lacked the ability to walk more than a hundred yards, hunching over like an old man, groaning with the pain increasing and shooting down my leg with each step. About five weeks earlier I was training at the gym one night after work and felt something, a pinch on the left side of my lower back. It was odd because the right side of my back had been finicky for over a decade, but never the left. Over the next week, I slowly lost the ability to stand upright or walk. The pain became excruciating. I stopped sleeping, unable to find a pain-free position. I spent the nighttime hours shifting positions every few minutes, riding wave after wave of pain-driven insomnia. By the end of the first week, I went to the doctor hoping to get an MRI because I knew this was a bad injury, but they said it was a pulled muscle and gave me a shot of Toradol, which is a strong pain reliever and anti-inflammatory. That didn't do jack. A few days later, I took a trip to the ER hoping to get an MRI, but my health insurance would not order it. I decided to pay out of pocket for an MRI to have peace of mind on what had happened. I wish that I hadn't.

The results came back. I had ruptured lumbar discs on both sides of my back between my fifth lumbar vertebrae and the sacrum, as well as bulging discs on each of the three levels above. I had an orthopedic surgeon look at my results and found several reasons for the pain. He suggested exploring surgical interventions. I declined. Having spent one year selling medical devices in Chicago, specifically spinal implants, I had learned very quickly that spine surgery is a last resort. I went with the rehab, wait, and hope route. I was confident that I could rehab myself. Judging from my current pain and immobility, that might take a while. Six months, maybe a year. I had faith the pain would be gone one day, and this outlook helped me through the darkest days when the pain was an 8 out of 10 during multiple concurrent sleepless nights.

I took a full four weeks off from Invictus and lay on my back on the floor at my house with my legs up on the bed. What a month! I was concerned that I was becoming a burden on Jess. She is independent to a fault and doesn't need me, often taking complete care of herself. I was worried that her care for me would run out. I couldn't walk, stand, or sleep, so that barred me from completing my household duties, namely shopping, cooking, and cleaning. I couldn't even cook breakfast for myself because frying up a few eggs took too long in the standing position, so I'd sit hunched in a mushy ball while cooking, or I'd eat something less nutritious that didn't require cooking. This was a big change from cooking every single meal that I ate. I loved cooking, and I missed it. By the end of that first four weeks, I could stand but not all the way up. I could walk, slouched. I could sleep, but most positions were painful the entire night. I had been injured many times in my life from sports and training, but this was by far the worst.

Lucky for me, Jess's patience lasted the full duration of my recovery. Prior to my back injury, Jess might cook once a week. Now, she was cooking almost every day. She brought me treats from work. She even grocery shopped, and she didn't complain. She did make fun of me, constantly. "Old man cripple, time to take your meds," she'd snark. We had been together for more than ten years, and she knew that I was really hurting. It melted my heart to see her taking care of me. I had not seen this tender side of her for more than fleeting instances over the last decade. This is when I first recognized what a wonderful mother she could be. One day, I hoped.

At home with Jess, all I could do was watch TV or play boardgames. Jess and I played Yahtzee. She won most of the time. When Jess was at work, I propped up pillows and blankets on the couch in the least painful position that I could find and watched Netflix with Snowflake sitting on my belly. She could sense my pain and seemed to mirror Jess's tenderness. She only growled at me occasionally.

Near the tail end of my month off from work, I got a call from Cam. She had just concluded the wildland fire season with the helitack crew and was ready to begin training again for smokejumper rookie training. My back pain was still debilitating, and the medication caused me to have a hard time controlling my emotions. On the phone with Cam, I tried as hard as I could to sound upbeat and vibrant. I didn't want her to sense my frailty and decide to train with someone else. After the past month of physical agony, this was a breath of fresh air. Cam was gunning for another shot.

In the fall of 2020 Cam 100% committed to working in Alaska. A large part of that was being close to Andy, but another big part of why she wanted to be an Alaska Smokejumper is because Alaska is an incredible place to work in aviation. She had persistently pursued jumping at the Bureau of Land Management's Fairbanks, Alaska smokejumper base, and they seemed more interested in her this year. They had noticed her persistence, dedication, and physical progress. Driven by hope for the future, I immediately began to feel better. Sometimes all it takes to push through a wall is a second chance.

MONDAY, NOVEMBER 23, 2020-SUNDAY, JANUARY 17, 2021 (TRAINING BLOCK ONE, 8 WEEKS)

Over the duration of the 2020 summer, in her mind, Cam had built rookie training up into a massive, scary beast. On the "GOALS" tab in her sheets, she wrote, "I wanted to take some time to write out a few goals before I get immersed in training. I think my biggest goal is to do some sort of breath work/ yoga/ meditation/ journaling every day. I have a lot of anxiety around Rookie Training already built up (more, I think, than last year) ... And I want to manage that in a healthy way, and not let it affect my training. As for physical goals, I hope to be able to do 18 pull ups, 100 push ups, and 150 sit ups. I want my 1.5 mi time to be consistently under 9 mins. I want to feel like a fast hiker too (part of that is actually getting fast, and part of that is feeling hecking strong and having confidence in my abilities)."

While reading this, I raised my eyebrows and nodded. Cam already seemed like a new athlete this year. The whole situation felt different. Despite admitting her anxiety, she seemed more poised. Her goals were now higher than last year, and she was committed to improving her mindset. I could not yet see any holes in her preparation pathway.

Week one, day one, amidst a lovely rendition of morning bass, I programmed her a PT test, same as last year, to see where she was. She had been training hard already, and I was looking forward to seeing her results. With her massive goals compared to last year already stated, I hoped to see some solid marks on her first PT test. She did not disappoint:

	BLM High Standards	*Cam's preseason scores*	*Cam's Initial Goals*
1.5-mile Run	9:30	9:50	9:00
Pull-ups	10	13	18
Push-ups	35	42	100
Sit-ups	60	83	150
Pack Test	110 lbs., 3 miles, 65 mins	no preseason test this year	110 lbs., 3 miles, 55 mins

This was an outstanding start. Already she was beyond the BLM high standards. During last year's training, her marks were not high enough to train towards completing some of the more rigorous training that I had in mind for her. This year would be different. I was now planning on progressing her faster and pushing her harder.

Her right hip and quad were still bothering her a bit after the wildland fire season, and her physical therapist had assigned some glute strengthening exercises. In her sheets, I wrote a place in each day for her to complete these important rehab tasks. I have found that athletes struggle with making time for physical therapy unless it's structured right into their daily training plan.

After the great PT test during week one, the rest of that week Cam completely crushed her training. Her recovery biofeedback was 5s across the board, her feedback in the sheets was complete and concise, and her attention to detail was sharp. I could feel the momentum.

In her spreadsheets, I added a tracking feature for weekly training time. At the top of each individual training day, I put a box there for Cam to type in her total training time in minutes, and I created a formula to add all those minutes up to calculate total work time for the week. This saved me a ton of time each week! In the past for Heidi, Sierra, and Cam last season, I was estimating and adding up training time manually. Now I put the power of tracking training time into Cam's hands.

Week one, Cam trained for a total of 13 hours, covered 21 miles of running and hiking, 100 pull-ups, 265 push-ups, and 430 reps of core training. Cam was back, stronger than ever. Compared to last year, Cam was months ahead.

During the first eight-week training block, Cam built from 40 to 65 pounds on the 3-mile heavy pack training, climbed from 21 to 30 weekly running and hiking miles, and peaked her weekly volume of pull-ups at 140 reps, 430 push-ups, and core training repetitions near 600. I also started her on a specific conditioning regimen to prepare her for Fairbanks rookie training, hitting multiple rounds of pull-ups, push-ups, sit-ups, and running. We were already far beyond where she had left off at the end of the last training season. I was impressed that Cam was able to train and improve throughout the summer fire season. That was unusual. In my limited experience coaching wildland fire athletes, during the summer months when wildfires are frequent, hitting consistent training sessions in addition to the physically demanding job as wildland firefighter is not easy. Cam was extremely dedicated. If last season she seemed to develop an obsession, this season she would perfect it. I felt that this was exactly what she needed to be successful at rookie training. The rookie trainers would push her to the edge, and she needed to drive her own edge out as far as humanly possible in the next four months.

Cam was living in Colorado, and snow was on the ground, so that meant backcountry skiing! Once again, this played many important roles in Cam's training as a fun task, trained her leg endurance and cardiorespiratory ability, and was good for mindset training through physically grinding for hours at one task. I loved this for her. She also began ice climbing again. The more "fun" opportunities that I could layer into her training schedule each week, the better, as long as they fit the training cycle, drove desirable adaptations, and weren't too dangerous.

At the end of the first block, Cam was already interviewing with smoke-jumper bases. Alaska seemed likely for the upcoming season, but it wasn't certain.

After those four weeks off from coaching, I went back to work at Invictus in early December. I had lost 20 pounds, now down to a sickly and frail 185 pounds, my lowest bodyweight since college, when I intentionally dropped 20 pounds over the course of two months during the end of my final collegiate track and field season, lightening my bodyweight to help me win the national championship in the long jump. I didn't like the way I looked then (even lost a girlfriend over it). And I didn't like the way I looked now.

Over the past month, I had to learn how to position myself in a way to allow sleep, and how to minimize pain while getting in and out of bed. How to cook for myself. Getting back into the swing of things at Invictus was tough. Demonstrating training drills for my athletes was out of the question for the first few weeks, and they understood. They noticed my striking physical transformation from healthy and vibrant to thin and broken. My athletes were worried about me. I assured them that I would heal completely. It would just take a while.

Now back at work, when at home on the weekends, the ornery miss Snowflake kept me company. We both growled at the tire shop when they played the bass too loud. We both limped outside to complain when the walls of the house shook. We had been spending a lot of time together. One morning while I was sitting hunched over at my desk, programming for my crew of athletes, Snow began to build a sandy line of cat litter across the light wooden floor. She must have taken a dozen potty visits all within an hour's time. I thought it was odd. She had never done this before. I thought she had a tough poop that she couldn't push out. Jess was still asleep, so I figured I'd wait to ask her what to do. I thought I heard Snow say in her English accent, "Bollocks. Me body ain't right."

When Jess woke up at eleven a.m. after her late-night work shift, she walked into the back office to see me sitting at my desk, hunched over, working away, and Snow in the corner of the litter box trying to squeeze out a pee. What is going on?! She's in pain! Look at her face!! We need to take her to the animal hospital right now. She is dying." I thought something not good was happening with Snow, but her dying was not on my mind. Jess's motherly instinct kicked in. She called our travel vet who agreed — Snow needed veterinary attention. Fortunately, it was a day off for both of us. We carefully put Snow in a cat crate and drove her to the animal hospital.

We learned two major things from the animal hospital. One, Snowflake was in fact a male cat. He simply had a tiny cat penis. Jess and I cracked up about this along with the vet tech who delivered the news, who said Snowflake "wasn't a proud boy." Apparently, it's common to mis-sex cats. Our travel vet couldn't find his penis. However, the second discovery at the animal hospital was not as funny. Snow had an infection in his urethra, giving us two options, surgery or euthanasia. When the nurse gave us our options, it seemed that she thought we would for-sure put Snowflake down. He was, after all, a beat-up old street cat with no canine teeth, horrendous breath, a British accent, and a temper. Growling, scratching, and cursing, he was always a terror at the vet, even when in pain. But for us, we were just getting to know and enjoy having him around the house. Jess and I looked into each other's eyes, and I knew we would keep him alive. We ponied up the money, and they did the surgery. He lived.

For the next few weeks, I had to give Snow his pills three times daily. Boy, that was something else. I was still in a fragile state from my back injury, and Snow had long sharp claws, and he was also in pain, so we had a helluva time getting those pills into his mouth. I brought back the old cat burrito trick from the bath days. When he wasn't looking, I'd sneak up behind him, wrap him up in a towel, careful to get all his crazy, clawed paws confined, and then we used a cat pill injection gun to shoot pills way down the back of his throat as he roared and growled and pierced his claws through the towel. I then had to physically hold his mouth shut, blow on his nose, and rub his throat to get him to swallow. We discovered if we didn't do it this way, he'd just wait a minute and then spit the pill back up. "Nice troy, ya pricks."

Ironically, now Snow and I were both on the same damn pills, a neurological agent that decreases nerve pain. What a scare. At least he was still alive. The vet said there was no way to know how much longer he'd live. As we recovered together, we bonded even more. He was now back to speaking with his angry old English man accent as he wobbled around the house like a milk drunk baby. I was still hobbling myself. We were quite the pair. After working at Invictus and doing my best to coach Olympic Weightlifting, I'd return home and finish programming for Cam and the other dozen athletes on my roster. Then I'd lie down on the couch, and Snow would curl up on my stomach and fall asleep. He made me feel like we were going to be ok.

MONDAY, JANUARY 18-SUNDAY, MARCH 14, 2021 (TRAINING BLOCK TWO, 8 WEEKS)

It had been about ten weeks since my back injury, and I was still recovering. I had gained my weight back, but it definitely wasn't muscle. Through the stress of throwing out my back and now Snow, Jess had also lost weight, and she didn't have much extra to lose. She looked too thin. My rehabilitation was mostly self-guided. I bought a book written by a trusted doctor and back expert on how to rehab an injured back and began following it to a T. I started with short duration planks, glute activation, and bracing. Everything irritated it a little bit, but the discomfort was tolerable. Many athletes experience some back pain through training and life, so I waded through my own recovery journey knowing that every single mistake and helpful discovery could be useful in coaching my current and future athletes.

Jess and I had been living in the little blue house in San Diego for just over three years. After too many months of noise from the tire shop at all hours of the day, we decided to move. The most difficult choice that we faced was whether to bring Snow with us. Sure, we had just dropped a ton of money to get his urethra fixed, but he had lived in the yard of the little blue house for his entire life, and we were afraid that moving him would be too stressful in his fragile state. After deliberating, we took the chance and brought him with us the short few miles to our new rental house.

I was concerned that I would throw my back out again during the move, but I simply worked carefully, bracing and lifting with intention. While we were loading up the truck in the alleyway, with the tire shop bass blasting, the owner of the business, a younger guy who was there seven days a week, walked over and asked us where we were moving to. Not far, I said, just over the freeway, and waved my arm in the general direction. He nodded, then asked why we were moving. I smiled, paused, and then told him it was because his music was too loud. We laughed together and he wished us well.

After loading up the truck, Jess and I said a quick farewell and thank you to our old place, packed Snowflake into a cat crate, and drove the mile and a half to our new house. We moved just down the road, but the neighborhood was much quieter. We lived on a dead-end street, so traffic was light. The house was a mustardy yellow with orange trim, two bedrooms, wood floors, and the old plaster walls that come with old houses. It was a bit larger than our last place, and we didn't share our lot with any other tenants. The neighbors seemed friendly, and there was a small park a short walk out our back door. We turned the car port into a gym, which was perfect for filming movement demonstrations, video coaching, and in-person coaching. Snowflake must have missed the old place more than we did. He had lived his entire life in that yard. We had only spent two and a half years there.

Cam's second training block was going well. In week one, she completed another PT test, moving her pull-ups to 14 (a lifetime best), push-ups to 51, and her sit-ups to 102 reps. She completed the 1.5-mile run in 9:32, her fastest run yet. It was the middle of January, and she was well on her way. However, she still lacked a candidate bid. She was growing anxious about not being accepted again this year. After working persistently last season and going away empty-handed, Cam was determined to train even harder. In the past, a few of her fellow hotshot crewmembers had attempted to become smokejumpers and hadn't made it. She knew that she would have to be smart about training, and that it would take more than just brute strength to make it through. Both dudes that she knew who had washed out of rookie training were super shredded and exceptionally fast runners.

She writes, "I was lucky enough to meet my husband after my first hotshot season, actually on a hiking trail in Rocky Mountain National Park. We fell in love really quickly that winter, but Andy worked as a commercial fisherman in Alaska. It felt like a world away at the time. Relationships and wildland fire could be a whole book in itself. The first day that I landed, I kept finding tears in my eyes because it was so incredibly beautiful. I knew right away that Alaska was a place that I wanted to be." And that was the final motivational piece. Cam's heart was in wildland fire, and she strongly desired to live in Alaska. What better way to do that than combining them? Smokejumping in Alaska.

She was already vastly stronger than last year, which was promising. During the first four weeks, we pushed Cam's running and hiking volume up to 49 miles a week for two weeks in a row. She also completed 160 pull-ups, 360 push-ups, and 690 core training repetitions in her third week, totaling over 20 hours of training. These numbers were comparable to her peak month from the previous season's training! During week four, I gave her a heavy deload. She was still consistently tracking her sleep, mood, and appetite, and ranked her appetite a 7! (out of 5). That's a great sign if training is going well. With heavy training volume, appetite should go up. If we push training volume up and appetite goes down, that's a sure sign of overreaching. While there is some benefit to chasing that strategy, it's a risky road. Her performances seemed to be improving steadily, so I kept her on the moderately aggressive yet safe route. Her sleep, recovery, and appetite feedback also backed up this choice. We were sitting in the sweet spot each week, pushing growth with what felt like minimal risk.

About halfway through the deload week, four weeks since the last test, it was time for Cam to perform another PT test. The night before, someone had tried to break into their house. She hadn't slept. For her test, Cam was on edge, having used up adrenaline in the middle of the night instead of getting restful sleep. I suggested she wait a day or two to test, but she wanted to see what she could do from a sleep-deprived and emotionally fatigued state:

- 15 pull-ups (lifetime best!)
- 58 push-ups (another lifetime best!!)
- 107 sit-ups (also her best performance!!!)
- 9:22 in the 1.5-mile (holy cow, she went 4 for 4 with PR's during this test. Amazing!)

This was the first time that Cam was happy with herself! I was relieved to see that the program continued to work well for her. If we kept up this rate of improvement, she would surely reach her PT score goals in the next few months.

I incorporated a new breathing drill for Cam, and she took to it well. To train her tolerance to the buildup of carbon dioxide in her blood, I had her perform breath hold walks once a week. To find out what level to start her at,

I had her perform a max distance exhale-hold walk and count her steps. The first time she completed this training, she took 25 steps. Next, she performed about 10 minutes of exhale-hold walking with 10–12 steps (40–50% of her max) before inhaling and starting the cycle over again. After a few weeks of this, she was gaining steps. I love this drill because it plays games with your mind. When CO2 levels increase in the blood, it can cause a feeling of anxiety, and with that comes anxious thoughts. Learning to relax and live with this feeling is a powerful mindset tool. Cam dug in each week. The breath hold walking was a new technique I learned from following Patrick McKeown, author of *The Oxygen Advantage*. From consuming his content, I learned many of the breathing protocols that I use with my athletes.

I didn't know about this specific breathwork drill when I had trained Heidi and Sierra. If I had, I would have used it with them as well.

Near the end of this block, we pushed Cam's training volume about ten percent higher than the peak of her previous mesocycle. During the peak week, she completed 200 pull-ups, 400 push-ups, almost 700 core movement reps, just shy of 50 miles of running, skiing, and hiking, totaling 20 hours of work. Her heavy pack training was at 90 pounds, which she completed in 55 minutes, faster than ever. And she could bang out a 300-rep core and glute finisher in 10–12 minutes and feel pretty good afterwards. My confidence with Cam's performance was beginning to soar.

Unprompted, Cam called me up one morning. A rarity. Of course, I was concerned. Through the phone, I could tell something good had happened. "Fritz, Alaska offered me a job!" I laughed and smiled big, congratulating her. It was a long time coming. After more than a full year of specific smokejumper training, Cam was offered a position at the Fairbanks, Alaska Smokejumper Base. Finally, we could train with full confidence. She would be attending rookie training in April, only two months away.

All first-time smokejumper job offers are contingent on passing rookie training. Cam was now past the first major hurdle to becoming a smokejumper, the application process. What a relief! For years she had worked on building her skills and experience to arrive at this point. As soon as I heard from Cam, I excitedly told Jess. Having listened to all my daily and weekly training recaps on how things were going with Cam, Jess was as invested in her story as I was.

Then things took a turn for the worse. During the peak week of the second training block, Cam performed a running workout with one of her future rookie bros and her quad began to feel irritated. When I read her feedback, my heart sank, and I felt a pang of energy well up in my abdomen. Cam's quad pain from last season was coming back to haunt her. While training her this season, my biggest fear was a recurrence of last year's nagging hip and quad injury. We had kept it at bay for months, but now it was beginning to rear its ugly head. I hoped to nip this in the bud before it got worse. I deloaded her heavily the next week, hoping that she would heal quickly. The volume and intensity of rookie training would expose this, potentially ending Cam's pursuit of smokejumper glory. We couldn't let that happen.

MONDAY, MARCH 15-SUNDAY, APRIL 4, 2021 (TRAINING BLOCK THREE, THE PEAK BLOCK! 3 WEEKS)

After the move, we kept Snow inside for a week to keep him from running back to the old place. There is no doubt that he could have found his way back. He seemed so much less stressed here. He acted sweeter towards us. I think that he was grateful to us for brining him. No more neighbor's cat outside in his territory getting him all riled up. No more clanging, banging, and loud bass shaking the house.

For the first few weeks, Snowflake seemed quite well until one day he wasn't. It only took about a month and then his health began to deteriorate rapidly. I thought he was going to be fine, but Jess thought he was dying. He began stumbling around and walking into things. We took him to the vet. Despite the expensive kidney diet that we had him on, his kidneys had failed, his blood pressure skyrocketed, and that caused him to go blind in a matter of days. Nothing could be done. After a few days of watching him struggle as he fell over and walked into things, we decided to put him down. We barely held it together when the euthanasia vet left our house with Snowflake's body gently wrapped in a blanket and placed into a wicker basket. Jess and I hugged each other and bawled our eyes out.

In the coming weeks, I missed Snow at my desk and in my lap. No more getting high together on the front porch. No more bath time. Even at the end, when he was blind and peeing on my lap as I held him, I missed that. The house still smelled like cat pee, and I was ok with that because it reminded me of him. I was dreading the day when all the remnants of him were gone. We assumed that cats live a long time, and we took his short time with us for granted. We had only had him for a couple of years. He was a street cat for most of his life, and that considerably shortened his life span. Even with his terrible breath, bad temper, and parasites, Snowflake had gently nuzzled his way into our hearts. We missed him greatly.

Despite my grief, I had work to do. Cam was entering the peak training block, and her quad was irritated. Just three short and crazy weeks of the highest volume training remained, followed by a three-week taper. I hoped that her body and mind would hold together. We could play it safe and complete a lighter training block, but I feared that setting the training volume too low here would risk her being washed in the first week. We were only six weeks away.

I specifically tightened training. More hiking with heavier packs, high volume PT, and more recovery skiing to help balance out her mindset. There's no use pushing all the way to her edge without an outlet, somewhere she could let off steam and enjoy herself, and skiing well served that purpose.

As exhilarating as the peak training block feels, it's also terrifying because you're pushing the athlete as close to the edge as possible. There is a ton of risk, and you must be on your game as coach and athlete, communicating clearly and immediately when things don't go as planned. Any little feeling or sensation in the body can be seen as a warning. Her quad issue from two weeks before was still present. I did not have complete confidence pushing her, but I knew that we had to. A sharp fear resided at the back of my mind, gently poking a needle of anxiety into my chest every so often, reminding me of the dangers, and what was at stake. I had pushed Heidi to the edge. Sierra, too. Now it was Cam's turn.

This is a graphic of Cam's peak training week:

	Monday	*Tuesday*	*Wednesday*	*Thursday*	*Friday*	*Saturday*
Running (miles)	Long slow distance	Intervals	**PT + Run**	**Intervals**	**Long slow distance**	**Fartlek**
	8.25	5	2.5	**5**	**10**	7
Hiking	Ski + sled pull		40 lbs.		100 lb. pack	
	5 miles		7 miles		3 miles	
Recovery (ski/fun)		RECOVERY	RECOVERY	RECOVERY	RECOVERY	RECOVERY
PT	Intensity		Heavy volume + Intensity		Light Volume	
Lower Body	Power Endurance		Volume Lunges	Bodyweight vol		Volume Lunges
Strength Accessory	Lower body		Lower + Upper		Upper body	
XPT Breathing	1. BOLT 2. Explore	Respiratory Muscle Training	Improve BOLT Walking Holds	CO2 Tolerance	Improve BOLT Walking Holds	Respiratory Muscle & CO2 Tolerance
Training (hours)	5 hours	3 hours	5 hours	3 hours	5 hours	3 hours

During this training block, Cam's weekly training duration hovered between 21 and 23 hours. Her total distance covered during the third and final peak week was 53 miles, comprised of 38 miles of running and 15 miles of hiking. One hike was a 3-hour ski while pulling a loaded sled over five miles. Cam's second hike that week sounded rough. She wrote, "7 mi, 180 mins, 2.6k vertical gain. Top was still snowy and muddy! 'Head down, keep moving.'"

I could hear her voice in my head as I read her feedback. The third hike was her final heavy pack training session which remained at 100 pounds throughout this three-week block. She had consistently clocked fast times.

One session during this training week was dedicated to bolstering high volume PT preparation. During week one, she completed a workout containing 70 pull-ups, 240 push-ups, 420 sit-ups, and two miles of 400-meter intervals. This took her 48 minutes and was a rough ride. She began to cramp in her hamstrings on the pull-ups, of all things. I imagined her curling her feet up behind her as she worked to squeeze out the final few reps of each set, and her hamstrings cramped in that position. We had a discussion afterwards about increasing hydration and electrolytes, specifically potassium, through her food. She mitigated this issue immediately and the cramping ceased. I used this high-volume PT session in week two as a slight deload and dropped her training volume and intensity. Even though this workout is no peach, in relation to the week before, it was easier, and she handled it well, shaving 16 minutes off her time. For the third and final week, I ramped the session up again, asking her to complete even more total work. She finished in just under 50 minutes and wrote, "hard push, but didn't  or cramp."

On this same training day, I wrote for her to complete as many rounds and repetitions as possible in 22 minutes of 120 abdominal, glute- and leg-strengthening tasks, 30 reps each. She completed 8 rounds. That's an average of 43 repetitions each minute, an unfathomable amount of core, glute, and leg muscle endurance. She knocked down similar tasks every day during the final peak week and logged a total of 190 pull-ups, 540 push-ups, and over 1,300 abdominal endurance repetitions across the six-day training week. Throughout this madness, her body held up.

During the peak block, Cam completed just enough strength training to maintain what she had built up to this point. I also wrote in a healthy serving of accessory work to keep her joints and tissues happy. She was diligent about spending time on body care after training. Serious full-time athletes honor this attention to detail despite the tedium, and in return, their bodies perform well for them. However, all the tissue work in the world cannot make an athlete bulletproof, especially when they are training near the edge of their capabilities. Cam was teetering on the edge. She woke up sore each day. Some days she was fatigued. Her joints were tender. Her muscles ached. She noted feeling her quad and IT band, but no pain. Just a warning to be careful. And when the body is sore and tired, mindset can begin to slip. Motivation can dry up. Some days she didn't want to get out of bed, but she did. All the physical discomfort and mental strain was a result of how far she had pushed her body and served as a clear reminder that she wasn't unbreakable. She was human. Cameron conquered her final peak week and now headed into the three-week taper towards Fairbanks day one.

MONDAY, APRIL 5-25, 2021
(THE FINAL TAPER, 3 WEEKS OUT)

It's about this time when athletes really begin to freak out about their upcoming event. Cam was no different. She was still nervous and had expressed anxiety about rookie training earlier this season. However, through experiencing a mountain of sheer physical work over the past five months, it seemed that every tough day she completed added resilience to her mindset. She was beginning to believe that passing rookie training was possible. In addition, I gave her my favorite pre-competition talk: the difference between nervous and excited. Feelings of excitement and nervousness are both composed of a similar hormonal cocktail. How an athlete chooses to frame this unique experience can massively impact how this normal and helpful physiological response to psychological stress feels. In addition, I explained that excitement is present to stimulate extra physiological output, meaning her body was preparing to access levels of performance that are not possible in lower stress states. The feeling is a good sign. It meant that her brain and body were aligning. It meant she was ready to go.

We had made it through the three peak training weeks unscathed. Cam was sore, tired, and on the edge of mentally quitting, but that's normal for the massive amount of physical work she had just completed. No major injuries except for one nagging quadricep and an irritated IT band, and we had successfully navigated around flaring them up any further through the past 60+ hours of training across three weeks. Finally, after months of hard training, hundreds of miles of running, hiking, skiing, and ice climbing, thousands of PT repetitions, accessory work, strength and power training, core bolstering, breath work, and mindset drills, we had arrived at the downhill slope of weekly training duration and volume. The end was in sight.

All that lay between Cam and her rookie training destiny in Fairbanks, Alaska, was a short three-week stint. We had passed the most stressful physical stage. Over the next three weeks, I planned to significantly decrease everything.

	Three Weeks Out	*Two Weeks Out*	*One Week Out*
Running	29 miles	23 miles	12 miles
Hiking	10 miles	9 miles	0 miles
Pull-ups	150 reps	120 reps	60 reps
Push-ups	450 reps	300 reps	150 reps
Core training	1000 reps	470 reps	200 reps
Training Hours	16 hours	8 hours	4 hours

The first taper week was a large decrease in training volume, bringing her training duration down to 16 hours from the 23 she had hit the week before. Cam ran 30 miles and hiked 10 for a total of 40 miles covered. She completed

155 pull-ups, 450 push-ups, and 1000 core reps. She also completed one final PT test and sent her data to Fairbanks. They were confident that she was physically ready.

	BLM High Standards	Cam's preseason scores	Cam's PT scores this week
1.5-mile Run	9:30	9:50	9:27
Pull-ups	10	13	15
Push-ups	35	42	62
Sit-ups	60	83	104
Pack Test	110 lbs., 3 miles, 65 mins	no preseason test this year	100 lbs., 3 miles, 58 mins

At the end of this week, she packed up and traveled to Fairbanks to get settled in for two weeks before the start of rookie training. Once Cam arrived in Alaska, she texted me an update on the situation. Due to Covid, she and the other rookies were assigned a 10-day quarantine from other humans. If she wasn't running or hiking alone, she was to be in her room. That meant training as well. She could not go to the gym. The rookie trainers were firm in their enforcement of this protocol. They didn't want anyone catching the virus and spreading it to the rest. They were about to embark on a five- to six-week journey together in close quarters and under heavy cardiorespiratory fatigue. The last thing any of them wanted was to catch a respiratory virus, rookie trainers included.

Taper week two was much less intense than week one. However, I wrote her one too many lunge-specific workouts and her quad began to act up. She mentioned it three times in her spreadsheets, and I simply missed it. By the time I viewed her feedback at the end of this week, she had skipped a handful of runs and hikes because her quad was bothering her. She had not skipped any training more than a single time up to this point. When I caught my error, it was too late. I called Cam up.

Me: "How are you doing?"

Cam: "Freaking out a bit. My quad, I can't use it. It feels crampy, locked up. What should I do?"

I broke out in a cold sweat. I knew this was a problem that required immediate attention. I could tell that Cam's confidence in her body was beginning to waver. It sounded like she needed a sports massage, but she couldn't see anyone in person due to the quarantine. I had been working with a specialist for my back rehabilitation and thought she might be able to help.

Me: "My body worker does remote consults. I'll put you in contact. She'll take care of you. We still have plenty of time to heal you up. You're still recovering from the high volume of those peak weeks, and you will heal up completely in the next two weeks."

Cam's voice changed. I could tell that seemed to give her hope. I hoped I was convincing enough. I knew the risks of sending an overtrained athlete into rookie training. If she showed up injured, she'd wash the first week. I didn't know if what I'd told her was true, but she needed to hear that her body was going to be ok. Without being able to push up to one hundred percent capacity, even the strongest mindset would not weather the physical storm that she was about to walk into.

That night, I contacted my specialist and she offered to perform a virtual assessment on Cam the next day. I paced back and forth, brow furrowed, teeth clenched together, wired, tired, and mind spinning. Months ago, Cam had heard through the grapevine that Fairbanks liked to smash their rookies with jumping lunges, so I had programmed a ton of them into her training. This had been a mistake. Let her hit a few here and there, but not so many that I ruin her on the home stretch. Had I helped Cam make it all this way to drop the ball 10 days out from rookie training? What was I thinking? What a waste. All that preparation down the drain. I had officially broken her. How was she supposed to run and hike and perform all the crazy things a week from now with a messed-up quad? It wasn't possible. That night I barely slept. Pavel would be disappointed in me.

The next day after Cam's session with my specialist, I called Cam and asked how she was doing. She said she "actually felt pretty good." A wave of sweet relief washed over me, dissolving the burning in my abdomen. Through a video session, the specialist taught Cam how to work out the knots in her quad. I was flabbergasted. I thought that Cam's quad was too far gone. Done. Cooked. I had seen athletes experience late season injuries before big competitions as a college athlete and while coaching at U of I. The athletic trainers do their best to mend them, and the athletes head into their season culmination event with a partially healed body and a mind teetering on the edge, confidence wavering, wondering if their body can obey what they must ask of it to surpass the team's and coach's expectations. Most of the time, the athlete would not push as hard as they could for lack of confidence in their body holding up, or if they were strong of mind and wanted to win badly enough, they would push to the edge, their body unable to hold up, and they'd further injure themselves. I had seen this many times. I wondered how Cam would hold up. I knew that she wasn't "fixed," but she was feeling better. That was an improvement for going into rookie training injured. We had one more week to go. I hoped that Cam would completely heal in time. I was positive with Cam, but deep down, I was very worried.

For her final week, I wrote in some PT reps, and some light accessory training that revolved around rehabbing her quad, or at least not irritating her further. Minimal hiking and running. On Friday, with three days to go, Cam tested out her quad. She wrote in the spreadsheets, "added in 3 x 10 banded jump squats, 10 walking lunges, and 10 jump lunges—all feels good!" A massive kettlebell was lifted off my chest. I took a deep breath and let it out slowly, relishing the short moment of serenity. When her quad held up, this was her sign that she was physically ready.

That weekend in her hotel room, I suggested that Cam complete the finishing touches on her mindset training by thinking about how far she had come. Reminiscing can be a powerful tool to increase the heart's desire, quell doubt, and summon gumption. In the past year and a half, Cameron had greatly improved, completing hundreds of training miles and thousands of PT repetitions. She had done everything in her power to put herself exactly here. It was time to show Fairbanks that they had made the right choice hiring her. And most importantly, it was time for her to meet her true self—the spirit that arises when the body and mind are maximally prepared and challenged.

MONDAY, APRIL 26, 2021 (ROOKIE TRAINING)

During Cam's first week, I waited eagerly for her to set massive new PT test PRs on day one, but the rookie trainers simply stopped each rookie once they had completed the bare minimum. That was the start of the mind games. It seemed like the rookie trainers were not letting them "eat." Letting the athletes eat is a phrase that old-timey coaches say when they are testing their athlete's output. Athletes love to test to see where they are, and even more, they love to complete against one another. Rookie training is no different. When you stop everyone at the minimums, it brings everyone to the same level. They all begin as equals, a team. And then the real work begins.

At the end of that first hellacious week, the rookie trainers tested maximum PT marks. Cam completed 16 pull-ups and 70 push-ups, both personal bests. I was happy to see the taper had worked, and she was able to improve her best marks even after a challenging and fatiguing first week, but I still wonder what she would have been able to produce if they had tested maxes when she was fresh on that first day. We'll never know.

All the pressure of training Cam was off my back. Now, the sensation was different. Waiting. I simply sat blind, anxious to hear how each week went. I needed a distraction, and what better way than a road trip up the scenic California Coast Highway. On a Friday afternoon, Jess had a long weekend off, so we packed overnight bags, hopped in the car, and drove north from San Diego. It was a light-hearted adventure with no plan. We didn't even have a hotel booked and figured we'd find a place along the way. The sun set a beautiful golden hue through the striated spring clouds as we casually cruised north, singing along to "Wonderwall" and "My Own Worst Enemy" and reminiscing about old times, talking about how far we had come and what our future might hold. A house. Kiddos. Growing old together. Getting more cats.

Jess asked about my athletes, and Cam was top of mind. How was she doing, we both wondered, and as if summoned, Cam's text came through. After completing week two, she was fatigued, sore, and still in the fight. I relaxed further back in my seat, rolled down the window, and smiled. "Good for her," Jess said, and stroked her fingernails along my forearm as it rested on the center console.

That night, we stayed in Port Hueneme, a small south-facing seaside town with a port and naval base. The next day, we woke up early and leisurely ate the hotel's continental breakfast, then hopped back on the 1 and continued northwards. It was an overcast and chilly morning along the coast. About an hour after hitting the road, we veered inland and the gray clouds parted, revealing a crystal blue sky and dazzling morning sun which illuminated the rich emerald and sage-colored grassy hills as our car climbed upwards. All the green and rolling terrain must have prompted an urge in Jess to wine taste, and just as she mentioned it, some billboards confirmed that wineries were close. We followed a road off the freeway further inland for a few miles, not knowing what we'd find. Soon enough, we began seeing simple white houses and buildings with clean, brown-lined wood zigzagging across them. We had stumbled into Solvang, a Southern Californian Danish-themed village famous for its architecture and wineries nestled in the Santa Ynez Valley. We had no idea the place existed.

The streets and businesses were bustling with tourists. We parked and walked the streets, eventually finding a wine tasting room and then a brewery. We drank too much and got a little buzzed, then walked it off around the town checking out the tourist shops before hopping back in the car. We drove further north to Morro Bay and booked another random motel for the night.

We arrived just before sundown and took a walk around the small town and ended up eating dinner at a little seaside restaurant called the Galley. We had some calamari and local fish. Jess ate the rockfish, and I had the king salmon. They were both delightful! That night back at our little motel, the people above us seemed to be dancing and moving furniture around all night. I woke up early the next morning on Sunday and went outside with my small travel laptop. I sat in the sun on a rickety old plastic chair and finished a good chunk of programming for my dozen athletes and noted that my work time was much shorter with Cam's preparation off my plate. Another smokejumper, here and gone. I felt a pang of melancholy as life momentarily slipped by more quickly than usual. I missed the challenge of getting all the details right on her programming, taking into context her last few weeks of training, and considering everything before tying it all together into her weekly plan. I texted her good luck for the upcoming third week of training. She was about to enter parachuting 101, the most technically demanding week. This is the week that Sierra was washed from Boise. I hoped Cam was physically fit enough to keep her mind focused on learning the landing technique and jump cadence.

On the Sunday drive home, my back flared up from all that time in the car. It took me a few days of stretching and bracing to reduce the discomfort. Even though six months had passed since my initial injury, I was still feeling the effects. I hoped one day the pain would cease for good.

Two more weeks passed, and at the end of each week, Cam checked in that she was still alive and kicking. I kept busy with coaching group classes at Invictus during the week, and on the weekend, programming for my growing crew of wildland fire athletes.

On a Tuesday, during Cam's sixth week of rookie training, she called me. I instantly felt a jolt of emotion. The call could be good or bad. It was too late for anything else. I took a breath, braced for impact, and hit the green accept button. "Fritz, I made it! I can't believe it's over. It was so ridiculously hard. The hardest thing I've ever done," she exclaimed.

I could tell by the waver and hoarseness in her voice that she was exhausted and excited and running on fumes. She thanked me for helping her prepare over the past two years. She said that she couldn't have done it without me. I thought that she probably could have but withheld my comment. I beamed and smiled from ear to ear. She had conquered the running, hiking, and all the PT. She overcame the jump tower. Days with 1000 push-ups. Days with 500 sit-ups in a single set, as a team. And in early May of 2021, after just over five weeks undergoing the most challenging physical training of her life, Cam graduated from rookie training with seven other rookie brothers who had battled the elements, elevation, and training together.

Out of the three smokejumpers that I had trained, I spent the most time preparing Cam—two full preparation seasons spanning a year and a half, and about 11 months spent working together as coach and athlete. During those two years of Cam's preparation, I relied heavily on Pavel's principles. I also leaned on what I had learned from Mike and Tonja for increasing Cam's running speed while keeping her feet and lower legs healthy and for tapering her smoothly into rookie training.

Out of all the athletes I had coached in my life, Cam had physically and mentally come the furthest. She had overcome her anxiety and cultivated a formidable mindset. She had blossomed into a physical specimen worthy of calling herself a smokejumper for the Bureau of Land Management in Fairbanks, Alaska. I was so proud of her. And I was close to proud of myself.

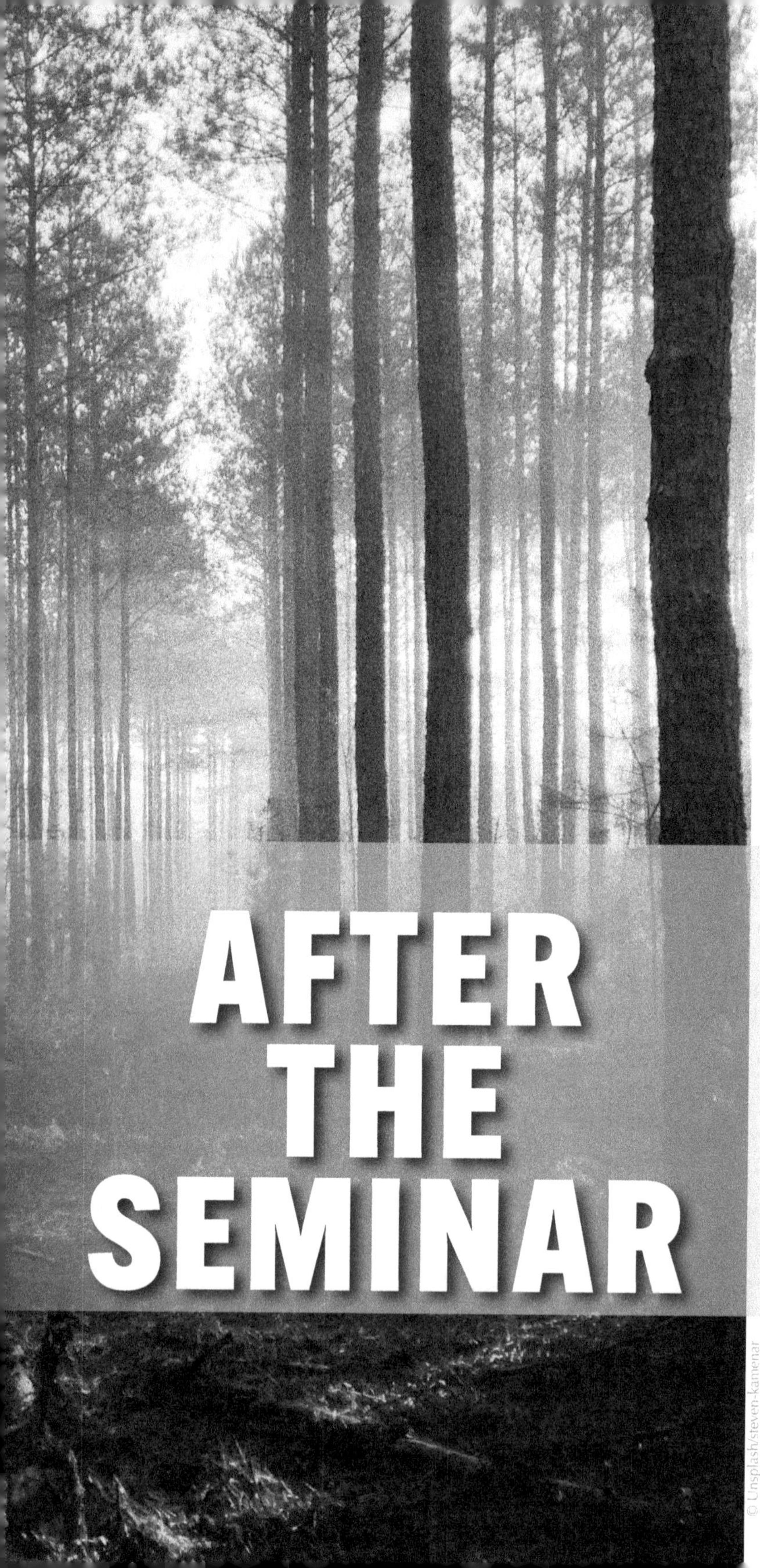

5 AFTER THE SEMINAR

WHILE I STOOD ON THE STAGE AT THE FRONT OF THE ROOM, EXPOSED, I FELT ENTIRELY VULNERABLE. I must have been up there half an hour or longer, drawing progressions on the white board and discussing my choices for training volumes and exercise selection. There were a few moments while standing opposite Pavel at the white board that I felt extreme pangs of imposter syndrome—a feeling when one's current situation is so far removed from what they think they are capable of that they feel like an outsider within their own skin. I had to consciously breathe slowly and deeply, and I kept telling myself that I was ok. *Keep your mind focused on the task. You're doing fine. No, don't drift up to the ceiling to hide. Stay here. You worked hard for this. No, don't play meek. They want to hear your story.*

Near the end of my stint on the stage, I began to feel more composed and fortunately glanced at some of the faces of the other coaches in the crowd. The females seemed to be taking rigorous notes, especially when I listed off the best marks for Heidi, Sierra, and Cam. The room was shocked to hear that Heidi had completed over 90 push-ups her first year during the smokejumper PT test. There was a gasp in the crowd from some of the women, who perhaps thought that was not possible. I momentarily questioned myself and set a mental note to double-check the data to make sure I wasn't overstating our accomplishments.

After a final discussion of my progressions and principles, I took some questions and eventually Pavel moved onto the next case study. I sat back down on the metal folding chair in the front row. A quiet disbelief settled over me. The seminar ended, and next, I had to get to the airport to fly back home. I felt the cool rush of the Colorado mountain air blow through the open-air gym as I gathered my things. While I packed up my things into my backpack, Pavel walked over to me, leaned down, and said, "I'm very interested to see your training progressions. What you did with these ladies is very impressive. Please send me your data." To anyone watching our interaction, it occurred quickly. I kept my composure, smiled, thanked him, and said that I would send him what I had. In my head, I was oozing with satisfaction. It had been more than twenty years since I had first seen him on the cover of the book that my mom had bought me in high school. In the span of an instant, I felt the magnitude of my life coming full circle, closing a giant loop.

I walked out of the gym down the back staircase and scheduled a Lyft to Denver International. As I waited for my ride in the shade of a building across the street, the magnitude of what had just occurred began to sink in. Heidi, Sierra, and Cam knew that we had done something special. We had accomplished a great feat preparing for one of the most challenging training processes in the United States. After sharing that experience at the seminar amongst the highest level of coaching critique, I experienced a validation of our efforts. I couldn't wait to share the news with the women.

On the plane, I pulled out my tiny travel computer and drafted an email to them, planning to send it off when we landed. In the email, I summarized my experience at the seminar and asked for all three women to send me their best testing marks from rookie training. I wanted to fact check what I said at the conference to ensure I wasn't exaggerating. Pavel is an intimidating figure, and I was quite nervous. When he presented at the conference, even though he effortlessly wielded deep knowledge and a dry wit, he still stoically joked at the beginning of the seminar that when on stage in front of a large group of people, one can only access partial intelligence, so I could always use this as an excuse if I had gotten my data wrong.

I got home from the airport just in time to see Jess before she left for work. I walked in and she greeted me with a kiss, asking how it went. I giddily began retelling the story about getting pulled up on stage to share about the smokejumpers. Jess said, "See, you know what you're doing!" I laughed it off, shaking my head, still in disbelief.

After she left, I found myself sitting in the back office, deep in thought. I sent the email off to the women, and then sat back, feet up on the desk, and exhaled deeply. I felt full of emotion, and I was uncertain what to do next.

For most of my life, I have felt that I wasn't good enough, wasn't worthy of the spotlight or success. I think this stems from a perfectionism that observes all actions and outcomes as short of optimal. If you're not the best, then you're not worthy of putting yourself and your ideas out there. This concept is flawed, of course.

I took some time to dig up Heidi, Sierra, and Cam's maximum PT marks to double check that my data was accurate at the conference. I had indeed gotten my data wrong. I realized that I had shorted Heidi's best push-up marks by over 20. I said her best score was 94 reps, which was close enough to her first season best mark of 95. Her second season as she trained for the perfect PT score, she had completed 118 push-ups. Sierra and Cam had each completed more than 70 reps. All three women had performed beyond what was thought possible at the conference. Then it all hit me at once. Before this, I had a feeling that what we had accomplished was challenging and rare, but I had no idea the magnitude of our success.

As I sat in an ergonomic swivel chair in my office, emotions that I had buried in the depths of myself began to well up to the surface. After each trainee's success, instead of fully celebrating and allowing joy to enter my heart, I had experienced self-doubt. Celebration stifled. This time, instead of resisting and pushing the emotions back down like I had many times throughout my life, I gave permission to the energy, and it rose until it flowed into my chest. As soon as it reached my heart, I began to cry. Continuing to sob, I involuntarily made my way to the floor and rolled up into the fetal position, letting it all release. Wave after wave of "you're not good enough," and "you're not fast enough," and "they'll never accept you" began to surface, each negative thought exploding into deeper sobbing as the joy from this weekend's experience shattered layers of negativity and self-contempt within me. I released a short lifetime's worth of pent up and deeply buried self-criticism and doubt. The emotional waves washed over me, and when the last one finally broke, I felt like a pile of boiled ramen noodles as I lay on my back. A contented smile crept across my face.

Within the next week, Heidi, Sierra, and Cam each sent me their PT data. I had not exaggerated and was relieved that I didn't speak loosely on the stage at the seminar. Once I had verified their data, I sent a lengthy email to Pavel with each of their best marks and how far they had come, as he had asked. After he received my email and data, he asked to see Heidi's 2018 programming. That was the training document from the year after Heidi made it through rookie training, the year that she attempted a run at a perfect 400-point PT score.

I sent Pavel the link to her training and warned him that it was in raw form and was not as streamlined as my current spreadsheets. It was nowhere near as organized and simple as Pavel's training programs. I was unsure what he wanted to see, but I was curious for his feedback and critique, and I told him so. We touched base over the next few months, but he never got around to critiquing Heidi's training. To make it up to me, he offered me free entry into a StrongFirst event—their all-terrain conditioning seminar. The course was geared towards preparing obstacle course racers, CrossFit athletes, fighters, first responders, and special operators (military and fire) to improve endurance and aerobic capacity. It was right up my alley. Upon receiving his offer, I realized, or at least I assumed what had happened. I imagine Pavel tried once or twice to sift through Heidi's training but was overwhelmed by the open format of my hundred-plus-lined spreadsheets with dozens of tabs and figured I needed some help simplifying my approach. He's a busy man and his time is precious. And he wasn't wrong. My programming style is immensely detailed and expansive, and within Heidi's spreadsheets, they border on chaotic. Even today I could still use some streamlining.

I took the course online because the event was taking place in two days in Seattle, and I couldn't swing the last-minute trip. Instead, I sat at my small particle board desk for sixteen hours during that weekend and scribbled enough notes to fill half a spiral bound notebook. I thoroughly enjoyed the seminar. It was a good refresher on the power of training easier and progressing slowly and intelligently. I also realized that many of my favorite drills and progression style for preparing smokejumpers for rookie training are similar to the methods taught by StrongFirst. I also realized that I would not be the coach I am today without Pavel's guidance from soaking up his knowledge through his books and live events over the past two decades. On Sunday night after the seminar ended, my heart was full, bursting with new inspiration as I programmed my athlete's training programs for the week.

• • •

Helping Heidi, Sierra, and Cam prepare for smokejumper rookie training was my most challenging and meaningful professional success. Through working with them, I learned and grew immensely. Now, as I look back through their training, it still blows my mind how much brutal, physical training I created for them. They each had their own burning reasons for staying the course. To this day, I still do not know what their deepest motivations were. It's probably best that way. Each of us must maintain a part of ourselves that is wholly our own.

At the beginning of each new wildland fire season, returning smokejumpers must retest their PT scores. The PT test acts as a motivator and benchmark for returning smokejumpers to show up fit and ready for the upcoming season. Matt Bowers, a retired smokejumper and crew supervisor at the Boise Smokejumper Base who worked with Heidi and Cam, and who also crossed paths with Sierra when she attended her first three weeks of rookie training at Boise, said they take the PT test seriously and incentivize progress each year by offering a paid day off if a smokejumper scores a mere 10 points higher than the previous year.

Matt and I spoke for a while. Near the end of our conversation, I asked him what type of person can become a smokejumper. He paused for a moment in reflection, then responded, "Well, anyone. The physical standards are within range for any human. They must want it bad enough." Not having considered this, I smiled, knowing that he was right.

The year after she passed rookie training at Boise, Heidi set her sights on returning that following season and putting up a perfect 400-point score on the PT test. Back to the drawing board at my desk I went. Heidi trained hard that off-season, and I pushed her as far as I could, again, but this time, we focused solely on hitting top PT marks. The training volume of hiking and running didn't need to be quite as high because the PT test was a single day and not a five-week rookie training selection, but the training was still immensely challenging. The volume was high, but the intensity near the end was like nothing I had ever pushed an athlete through before. Heidi's boyfriend, who was also a wildland firefighter, complained that she trained too much.

	BLM 100-point Targets	***Heidi's 2018 Marks***	***Score***
1.5-mile Run	8:00	9:45	46 points
Pull-ups	25	25 (dead-on)	100 points
Push-ups	120	118 (2 short)	99 points
Sit-ups	150	148 (2 short)	99 points
		Total:	344 points

For Heidi to score a perfect 400 points, she would have to complete 25 strict pull-ups, 120 push-ups, 150 sit-ups, and run the 1.5-mile in a blisteringly fast 8:00, which comes out to a 5:20 mile pace. After battling through setbacks and nagging injuries, she showed up and completed 25 pull-ups (100 points!), 118 push-ups (99 points), and 148 sit-ups (99 points). When she got to the 1.5-mile run, after a full season of battling plantar fasciitis, she ruptured her plantar fascia at the bottom of her foot and ended up finishing around 9:45 (lower points than she had hoped). We both did our best and she came up short. I'm still proud of her marks, though. They remain the highest PT scores of anyone I have ever coached, male or female.

That was five years ago. Since then, after each fire season in November or December, Heidi contacts me to start up her training. The goal each year is to crush the pre-fire season PT test and prepare her for the demands of wildland fire. She is no longer a smokejumper. After four seasons smoke jumping in Boise, she is now a hotshot squad boss in Bishop, California. She turns 40 this year and still trains like a 25-year-old. She is truly an amazing human, and I am grateful to continue training her after all these years.

I began coaching her again this year. We hopped on a phone call a few weeks ago to iron out the details of her training plan for the upcoming wildland fire preseason. Heidi informed me that, for the first time, the Bureau of Land Management changed the PT standards. They split the male and female standards, and the female standards are significantly lower.

Pull-Up Repetitions			*Push-Up Repetitions*			*1.5-mile Run Time*		
Males	**Points**	**Females**	**Males**	**Points**	**Females**	**Males**	**Points**	**Females**
25	100	15	120	100	70	8:00	100	9:00
	99		118	99	69	8:02	99	9:02
24	98		117	98	68	8:04	98	9:04
	97		115	97	67	8:05	97	9:05
	96		113	96	66	8:07	96	9:07
	95		112	95	65	8:09	95	9:09
23	94	14	110	94	64	8:11	94	9:11

Heidi thinks this isn't good for wildland fire. I agree. While on a fire assignment, women are expected to perform the same professional and physical duties as males. The PT standards should be equal as well. However, from this split in standards, it seems that the BLM holds women as physically less capable than their male colleagues. Perhaps they lowered the standards to increase accessibility to wildland firefighting to more females. Each year, the number of wildland firefighters decreases. Bowers attributes this to the growing number of other comparably similar-paying jobs which are much less physically demanding and don't require employees to be away from their families for weeks to months at a time. In addition, I attribute the decrease to the backsliding of the average health of the American populace. As our country becomes more overweight and obese, the percentage of able-bodied humans to fill wildland fire positions diminishes every year.

While I respect the BLM's outreach to enable more women into the wildland fire realm, I believe that the physical standards should remain equal. Inequality is potentially dangerous. Imagine working with a colleague who is less physically fit than you. Will you have to do more work? Will you have to pick up their slack? Will you have to physically carry them out of a rough situation? You are getting paid the same, and they won't be asked to do as much physically taxing work as you. I can imagine this type of inequality would quickly challenge team camaraderie.

Even though I disagree with the separation of male and female standards, it's rewarding to see where Heidi, Sierra, and Cam each stacked up. Against the new female scoring tables, Sierra and Cam would have scored either a perfect 400 points, or damn close. Heidi would have obliterated those standards.

It's been a breath of fresh air to reconnect with Heidi beyond training. To write this book, we hopped on phone calls, texted, and emailed back and forth. At her request, I sent an early version of the Heidi chapter for her to edit. Her feedback within the edits, as always, was heartfelt and thorough. While training Heidi, I referred to rookie training as "camp." I'm not sure how that started, but she thought it was cute and didn't correct me, hence the name "camp abs," which really means "rookie training abs." I must have imagined her at rookie training camp. I still had this misconception when I wrote the first draft of Heidi's chapter. When she read through it, she changed every single instance of "camp" to "rookie training." There were more than 100 corrections on that alone. That's how much this book means to her. She wants me to sound as credible as possible so we can reach a large audience and positively influence wildland fire.

Throughout this process, I learned more about Heidi's backstory. I finally asked why she chose me. She wrote back, "Haha this call, to me, it felt like I was calling the man who was going to clear up all my problems! I just handed you a pile and somehow I knew you could sort it out. I had 100% trust in you. And I knew whatever you told me to do, I would do."

While she edited, Heidi loved rereading her old visualizations. She had forgotten them. She writes, "Fritz! This is so special. This is so cool! I love this. Thank you for writing this book. I will cherish it forever. It is fun and funny to look back on things I said."

When referring to one of her visualizations that I quoted in her chapter, she writes, "I also like how I would include my rookie bros to be and even brought them into my positive thinking, that we all got it!" Heidi was such a strong team player that even in her visualizations, she included other teammates in her success. This is what makes her such an amazing leader and wildland firefighter. She's not in it for herself alone. She seems to live by the mindset that we're all in this together.

One last Heidi quote before I move on. When editing the book and rereading her old visualizations, she realized how sharp she used to be. She writes, "I love this, I am so happy you have included these in the chapter. I'm reminiscing on the past and makes me feel weak now." I am empathetic to her feelings on this. Having been a high-performing athlete years ago, I responded, "There is no need for our bodies and minds to maintain this level of mental fortitude. It takes too much energy. We all fall off the tip of the spear eventually. At least you had your success on top. Most people never experience the raw power and beauty of their full human potential."

Perhaps the thing that I cherish most about Heidi is the confidence which she instills in others, and this is directly tied to her "we is greater than me" mentality. Recently, I picked up a wildland fire athlete who had been selected into rappelling rookie training. Heidi had pointed her in my direction. When I spoke to this young woman on the phone, she mentioned how anxious she was for her upcoming rookie training (she came to me with six weeks to go, which is cutting it close, to put it mildly), and after speaking with Heidi, her nerves had calmed. She also described Heidi as a rig and a unit. I laughed and cracked a genuine smile and told her that Heidi had just turned 40.

A ***rig*** or ***unit*** is a person that looks like a titanium brick with human features. Pure muscle. A physical specimen. Formidable. Infinitely capable.

When I have difficulty keeping an athlete focused on their training program, I call in the big guns, and Heidi hops on the phone and helps them get their head right. She has a bear trap of a mind, so potent that a single conversation with her can put even the most anxious wildland firefighters at ease.

Heidi continues to lead in wildland fire, and I look forward to many more years of working in conjunction with her to help prepare more young and talented humans for the physical demands of wildland fire.

• • •

Sierra was my most challenging smokejumper. As with Heidi and Cam, I learned Sierra's backstory while writing this book. She was initially driven to become a wildland firefighter soon after finishing her undergraduate degree, "Because I desperately needed a job after college and someone in my geography program said they had done it and it was just like camping and hiking in the woods. Wow—I can get paid to hike and camp? I'm in! I honestly didn't care much about the 'fire' part of it. I loved that job and did it for another 12 years when I decided I better do something where I get paid more and have a pension—hence the city fire. Never quite my passion although there are aspects I enjoy," she wrote.

I was also curious to learn more about Sierra. I asked her about how she got into endurance running and what she likes about ultrarunning. She responded, "As far as the endurance stuff—I was exposed to it pretty young as my dad and brother were running 100s years before I even thought about it. I did a lot of running and endurance hikes with my dad and brother (especially in the Grand Canyon having grown up in Flagstaff) over the years and eventually it ended a passion of my own. When I ask myself the question Why run 100 miles?, I often think it's a bit of a waste of time, and it's horrendously painful (as I have injuries) but it's also somewhat instinctual and obviously therapeutic. It's a lot of time to 'work out your problems!' But is it just a distraction from real life? I do enjoy that it starts a conversation about what we do with our time. To one person it's crazy to run 100 miles, to another it's crazy to watch TV all day. I wouldn't say either one are necessarily productive, but I would say that I just really love to be in motion, and I love to test the limits of my body, and I love exploring the experience of the mind body soul connection—this includes dealing with pain and exploring pain. I think it puts certain aspects of life into perspective. In this way it is also spiritual. Mostly I love the trails and being In beautiful places!"

Sierra was a smokejumper at Redmond for one season. At the end of her rookie season, she landed badly on a training jump and fractured her hip. After multiple surgeries across many months, the doctor ended up shaving off her teres ligament, the root piece of connective tissue that connects the femoral head into the hip socket. Following the series of surgeries, Sierra could not walk for some time. The doctor told her that she may never run again. This was hard news for Sierra as she had been a runner for her entire life, and much of her identity is interwoven with the freedom of running through the mountains along a narrow and treacherous trail for miles and hours on end. When she called me to ask what I thought, I asked her what she wanted to do about it. She said she wanted to run ultras again. Of course, she did! I said let's get your strength back up and see what happens. Fast forward a few years, and Sierra is now back to running ultramarathons once again. This past fall, she competed in a 50-miler through the Arizona backcountry called, "Man vs. Horse." I'm currently training her for the Zion 100-miler in April of 2023. In the last three weeks, she has run over 225 miles. She wants to place top five, but I think she has a chance to win it.

At 43 years of age, Sierra recently finished her yearly PT test for San Diego fire where she broke the all-time female record for the treadmill VO2 max test. She still takes long spear-fishing trips to Mexico, and the wine bottle wall in her house is complete. Sierra and I still maintain a coaching relationship in the off-season, and our connection is strong. She follows what I write for her (most of the time). Years ago, if Sierra and I had failed, this book would not exist, and my blossoming wildland fire coaching career would not have continued. Luckily for me, Sierra is a specimen. I am grateful that she chose me to help her.

• • •

Cam lives in Fairbanks, Alaska, and recently eloped with Andy. She exudes contentment with her life, and it warms my heart. Last year, she finished her second season of smokejumping out of AK (Fairbanks, Alaska. She abbreviates it as AK). She loves her job and says she's not that good at it, yet. When she told me this, I laughed at the complexity of her statement and wondered how long it takes someone to become good at jumping out of a plane and aiming for their landing zone which might be a small clearing surrounded by tall trees on the side of a mountain. When you imagine this in your mind, make sure to factor in wind and a forest fire somewhere close by, and sprinkle in a healthy serving of excitement, fear, and the very real mortal danger.

While writing her chapter, I realized just how little I knew about the illusive Cameron. My editors constantly asked me, "Who is Cam? What's she about?" I was embarrassed by how little I knew about this woman that I had trained for almost two years. Like my work with Heidi and Sierra, I focused on the nuts and bolts of her daily preparation, how she was recovering, and how to squeeze every ounce of performance out of her before rookie training.

After being prompted by my editors to dig into Cam's story, I realized how intriguing it is—like something out of a western-action-romance-fiction novel. The part in her chapter about working in Rocky Mountain National Park was gathered years later during the creation of this book. Even more reason for me to be grateful for having written this. I was *forced* to get to know these wonderful women that I knew rather well in one aspect and remained wholly unacquainted in another for years.

At first, Cam was reluctant to allow me to write about her, knowing that even if I used a pseudonym for her, she is the only female jumper at Alaska for over a decade. It would be easy for someone to figure out who she is. At Heidi's behest, I spoke to Matt Bowers and after relaying to Cam that he was excited for this book to potentially help drive more people (and women) into wildland fire, she realized that her story was worth sharing and could help promote growth in her industry.

Here's what she wrote:

> *I started with 10 total in my rookie class. 8 made it through, including me. No other female rookie candidates in my year. And I am still the only lady jumping in Alaska (out of 75 total). I don't think there were any female candidates for the BLM last year. And I know there isn't one at least for Alaska this year. The last time a woman made it through rookie training in AK before me was in 2008. It really surprises me because I feel like it's an awesome place to work, and there are quite a few strong women that work in fire in Alaska in general. I just don't think very many qualified female applicants apply and take the application process seriously. Hopefully your book helps inspire a few more lady jumpers!*

Another big part of why I wanted to be an Alaska Smokejumper is because Alaska is an incredible place to work in aviation. The state is so big that airplane (and parachute) is the best way to access some of the most remote places. Often, there are no signs of human habitation anywhere around the places that we jump in to. We typically protect native allotments (used for subsistence hunting and trapping), remote homesteads and trapper cabins, historic sites and ecologically sensitive regions (like critical habitat for sensitive species), and remote villages. I love getting to go to places that are so far off of the road system. We cover fires in an area that is about as big as the whole Western continental United States. Sometimes we fly for 3 hours in a small commuter jet (a DHC-8) to jump a fire. This past season, I went to the Aleutian Islands, dunked my head in the Bering Sea, did project work among the Brown Bears of Katmai National Park (a highlight of my entire life, they are amazing creatures to see), spent 10 days protecting a trapline at the foot of the Brooks Range, and saw thousands of walruses from the plane. It's really hard to find the right words for how adventurous and cool it can be to get to jump into these super remote places under the midnight sun. Alaskan summer is a drug like no other ...

Recently, she texted me some helmet camera videos of her parachuting. She asked me not to share them. She writes, "I ask that you not share them because my flying isn't perfect in any of the videos that I have. I can never seem to record my best jumps for some reason ..." I laughed at this and loved watching the videos. I watched her transition from sitting in the doorway of the plane with her feet hanging out, tension building as the clouds whipped by at 95 knots, my heart jumping as she pushed out of the plane and shot downwards to the landing zone, a clearing in the middle of a forest, all within a minute and a half. She landed right between a pile of her smokejumper crewmates, and the video cuts out with them complimenting Cam on her accuracy (she almost landed on top of them).

Verifying her skill and character, Matt Bowers jumped with Cam on his very last roll as a smokejumper before retiring last year. He said that Cam was super strong, hardworking, had a great attitude, and added that she's an excellent smokejumper. Part of the reason that Cam allowed me to include her chapter in this book was because Matt (and Heidi) thought it might help get more females into wildland fire.

Parachuting as a smokejumper is different than recreational skydiving, and over the break between the 2022 and 2023 seasons, Cam learned to recreationally skydive. She wrote:

Getting my A License was awesome! It was 25 jumps. The first 7 jumps were super specific skills with 1 or 2 instructors, just working on the basics of free fall and canopy flight. At first, it was a challenge to get out of the airplane, but after a few jumps, I was totally captivated by the feeling of free fall. I will send you a video of one of my jumps. It is such an incredible sensation to push off the air and float around in the sky for over a minute! I did 10 more jumps after I got my license and got up to all kinds of shenanigans—flips out of the plane, rolling out backwards, grabbing another person's ankles and rolling out in a big somersault, jumping out with 8 people and making shapes (a star, a zipper) during free fall, flying like superman as far as I could go. It was really a cool experience. It won't translate very much to being a smokejumper, but I think it will help me a lot to overcome some of my stress getting out of the door of the aircraft. And it was so cool to just have fun and enjoy flying, rather than having to focus so much on doing all of my procedures perfectly. It's so amazing to be alive in a time when humans get to jump out of airplanes for fun and experience the magic of flight. I will definitely be doing more skydiving! It does feel a little hard to turn my focus to smokejumping again. It's still really really cold and snowy in Fairbanks. It was -20 when I landed here. But summer comes fast! And I will be flying again soon to super cool places.

Cam had one major request for this book: that I reveal minimal details about rookie training. She believes the process must be a surprise for rookies, and I tend to agree. There are traditional elements to each smokejumper base's rookie training, and other physical tests that are unique to the rookie trainers that lead the training. I hope that I didn't give away too much. And even if I did, good luck. To become a smokejumper, you'll need all the luck you can get, a trustworthy training program, and relentless grit.

• • •

Success with Heidi, Sierra, and Cam has generated more coaching opportunities for me with wildland fire athletes. Nowadays, when I speak with wildland hopefuls interested in making a run at a hotshot crew, helitack, rappelling, or smokejumping, they seem more eager to listen and trust me. It must be a combination of the quality referrals, my speaking with heightened confidence, better use of industry lingo, and a stronger belief that my programming works and is worthy of their consideration.

When people ask me about what I helped Heidi, Sierra, and Cameron accomplish, I explain that I tried to balance their hard work with my support. It wasn't all them (85%), and it certainly wasn't all me, either (~15%). It was a team effort. Perhaps most notably, after my psychological release of all that pent up negativity, life has been smooth as a spring breeze.

During the winter and spring of 2022, I prepared my first male smokejumper for rookie training. His name was Johnny. He heard about my programming through Cam. Before starting him on the program, I asked him to send me an injury list so I could troubleshoot and create his season preparation outline. He was an extreme snowboarder and sent me an injury summary almost three single-spaced pages in length. Over the next twelve weeks, I guided him through a periodic progression to produce what felt like the finest smokejumper physical preparation that I had been a part of. His injuries did not hinder him during rookie training, which is remarkable.

After he passed, I debriefed about him with Heidi. She wasn't surprised. "If you can supercharge an athlete my size, of course your program will create an absolute beast out of a 180-pound guy like Johnny," she chimed. Johnny crushed the selection process. I had learned so much from coaching Heidi, Sierra, and Cam, that the year coaching him went smooth as butter. No hiccups. That's a rarity with the physical preparation of any athlete, especially one peaking 25+ training hours a month out from selection. I'm sure that our training experience was no peach for him, though. I pushed him as hard as I had pushed anyone.

Johnny told me that one of the other rookies from his class, Luke, had washed out and spent a few days in the hospital afterwards. Luke wanted to speak with me to hear how Johnny and I trained to produce what seemed like a weapon of a wildland firefighter. According to Luke and other rookies in their class, he seemed to have an easy time. Eventually, I called Johnny to catch up and asked him if rookie training was easy for him. He chuckled and firmly denied it, saying rookie training was the most difficult physical, mental, and emotional challenge of his life and he would not elect to undergo it again.

Either way, I took this as a compliment and testament to the soundness of our preparation strategy. From Johnny's vantage point, he worked as hard as he could, and rookie training was the ultimate physical and mental challenge. To the other rookies, it seemed easy for him. I will be training Luke this season to prepare him for his old hotshot crew in the upcoming 2023 season. He won't be attempting smokejumper rookie training this year. He needs another year to heal from last year. Maybe he'll take another shot at rookie training in the spring of 2024.

In addition to training Luke, I was put in contact with an additional rookie candidate, Jeremy, another one of Johnny's colleagues. Jeremy is slated to tackle rappelling rookie training in April 2023. This is a form of Helitack, dropping crews off at wildfire sites where they rappel down from the helicopter to limit the spread of wildfires or rappel down cliff faces to reach wildfires in locations that smokejumpers may not be able to parachute into safely. I heard through the grapevine the selection process for this crew is tough, almost as tough as smokejumper selection. Once again, I'm excited to be a part of another rookie's preparation journey. Helping these athletes is a joyful experience. I am maximally challenged and fully engaged and do everything I can to help them succeed. I might even go as far as to say that coaching wildland fire athletes is my calling, and oddly enough, one completely delivered by fate. I would have never sought this pathway out without Heidi coming to me many years ago. My gratitude to her is immense.

My back still bothers me from time to time, but luckily, I found a new coach to take over my training, Jessica. I follow her program, and she coaches me, keeping my ego in check. "That's too heavy. Take some weight off," she might warn. I whine, "Awe, come on, coach! It's been over a week since my last injury!" Fortunately, I have steadily progressed without setback since my back injury, but I have hurt myself enough times in my life that she laughs. I make a pouty face and take the weight back down. Nowadays, I choose to prepare others for challenging tasks and live vicariously through their experiences and triumphs. I had my time in the sun as an athlete. Today, it's safe to say my competition days are behind me.

Perhaps most exciting, Jess is pregnant and due in March. During her pregnancy, we decided to learn the sex of the baby. I thought it would be fun to hit something for the gender reveal, so I had a friend load up a pumpkin piñata (it was late October) with pink or blue taffy. After smashing that pumpkin with a crowbar, I watched helplessly as pink taffy spilled downwards all over my deck, instantly signifying that we were having a girl. "What am I going to do with a girl?!" I exclaimed. I had grown up with my mom, dad, and my younger brother, so the house was a boy's paradise.

In 2022, Heidi recommended me to another smokejumper hopeful. One day, while speaking on the phone with this young woman, I paced back and forth in my garden as the sun warmed my skin and my bare feet sank into the sandy soil and told her about my encounter at the seminar with Pavel and his top coaches. Her response was the final straw on the camel's back when she demanded that I write this book. She said in the world of wildland fire, women have been performing at the elite level for decades, and in other highly physical realms, women are not well represented. She attributed this to females being unaware of the elite physical potential of their bodies, perhaps because they have been told they are incapable and inferior for so long that they believe it.

I asked her why she felt this way. She responded, "I grew up in a small town with some extreme and strong female role models who were wildland firefighters, so it was very clear to me from a young age the capacity for the female body was nearly limitless, and that fighting forest fires in the remote backcountry was not off limits for me or any other woman willing to work hard enough to earn it."

I found this a raw and beautiful example that exposure at a young age to something powerful can facilitate self-belief deep enough to completely override societal norms and the sentiments of those who might say, "It's not possible" and "That hasn't been done before." When you have seen someone who looks like you do what others say is impossible, an unshakable seed of belief is planted and remains at the core of who you are.

After a few months of thinking about what I should do with my daughter, the answer to that question has become clearer, although I cannot yet picture myself a parent. Raise her to be a competent, confident, and strong person.

Set a good example for her to see the value of physical health by training regularly and inviting her to watch and eventually join the training experience. She doesn't have to become a wildland firefighter, of course, but if she decided to go that route, I might know someone who could help her prepare. Most importantly, I desire for her to choose her own path and to walk it without the hindrance of self-doubt in her ability or potential simply because she was born a woman. Hopefully her exposure to strong female role models like Jess and the other elite women that I train will instill in her a drive to challenge herself and strive to live with passion and meaning in whatever realm she chooses.

GLOSSARY

TERM	DEFINITION
ACTIVE RECOVERY	Active recovery refers to low-intensity exercise or movement performed during the rest or recovery period between higher intensity or higher volume training days and aids in the recovery process by increasing blood flow to the muscles, reducing muscle soreness and stiffness, and stimulating the removal of metabolic waste products.
BACKCOUNTRY SKIN	Skinning is attaching synthetic "skins" onto the bottom of cross country skis to increase grip while hiking up a mountain to ski down the backcountry. Backcountry refers to remote and undeveloped areas, often outside of designated trails or resorts, that are typically accessed by hiking, skiing, or other outdoor activities. These areas are often characterized by rugged terrain, limited access to amenities, and a higher degree of risk and self-sufficiency than more developed areas.
BREATH HOLD WALKS	Breath hold walks are an advanced method to increase carbon dioxide (CO2) tolerance. When we breathe in oxygen to produce energy for performing all cellular actions, CO2 is produced as a byproduct. Increasing rates of CO2 buildup accompany higher exercise outputs. Building tolerance to increasing CO2 levels is helpful to mitigate or acclimate to the effects of high intensity exercise, altitude exposure, and psychological stress, all things wildland firefighters will encounter.
CAMP ABS	"Hello dollies" and "Flutter kicks" are two infamous core smashing drills that the women experienced in preparation for rookie training.
DECATHLON	An athletic event in the sport of track and field and takes place over two days. Each competitor takes part in ten events (100-meter dash, long jump, shot put, high jump, 400-meter dash, 110-meter hurdles, discus, pole vault, javelin, and 1,500-meter run).
DELOAD	A deload is a lighter volume and/or intensity stretch of time which allows the athlete to recover and prepare for the next increase in training volume and/or intensity. A single deload week is common during heavy training, and multiple consecutive deload weeks can be useful in the off-season to stimulate full recovery of the athlete's bodily systems.

DETRAINING	Detraining occurs when an athlete stops training or decreases training volume, intensity, or both, over a period longer than a few weeks to a few months, or longer. For wildland firefighters, this often occurs during fire season, and by the end of the season, they are in a detrained state. Physically, they are incapable of performing at the capacity they had when they entered the season.
DROP SETS	Drop sets in exercise refer to a technique where the athlete performs a set of an exercise until they reach muscle fatigue, and then immediately reduces the weight or repetitions and continues with another set with incomplete rest. This is typically done for multiple "drops" or reductions of resistance or repetitions in the same set to achieve muscle exhaustion and promote hypertrophy (muscle growth). This technique is often used to break through plateaus and challenge the muscles in new ways.
ESRI	Esri is an American multinational geographic information system (GIS) software company. Esri is the world's leading supplier of GIS software, web GIS, and geodatabase management applications. The company is headquartered in Redlands, California.
FARTLEK TRAINING	Fartlek runs are a form of interval training. This type of running workout is traditionally unstructured, meaning the parameters for how to perform the intervals can be loose and flexible. For example, over a 2-5-mile distance, for interval parameters, I may have athletes: • Use time—30 seconds run a bit faster + 60 seconds recovery pace • Use distances—100 meters push pace + 300 meters easy recovery jog • Use unique, flexible distances—Run fast to the next telephone pole + slow recovery jog to the following pole • Strides—30 hard strides + 50 easy-paced strides (A stride is left-right, every other step. Strides are easier to count than steps.) • And even breathing—Run hard for 10 full breath cycles + easy run for 25 slow recovery breaths The parameters are limited by landscape, the athlete's unique preferences and abilities, and the creativity of the coach!

FLOW	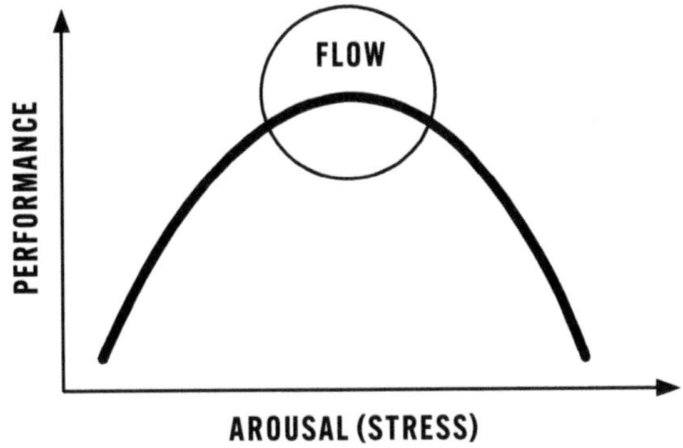 Toggling between sympathetic and parasympathetic stimulation in real time, right on the keystone, is a state referred to as flow. Flow is the most useful state for athletes (and humans, I argue) because here we precariously dance atop the performance arousal arch, living in the moment. This is where performance in anything that requires high cognitive, fine motor skill, or the blending of the two, is maximized. The concept of "flow" is the feeling of losing oneself in the moment. Flow is a desirable state for creatives like musicians, artists, and athletes. One cannot summon flow. You can set the stage for it, but flow must find you. As soon as you notice that you're in flow, you are no longer in flow because you are now noticing and not experiencing. A good personal example of this—I love to hike up a mountain trail and then run it back down. I wear those weird toe shoes, and they don't have much of a sole, so I feel every bit of texture on the trail. If I step on a rock, it hurts. When I run down the mountain, I must watch exactly where I place each footstep, to the centimeter. If I think "step there, there, and there," I will slip or fall or step on a sharp rock. I won't move as quickly compared to when I turn off my thinking brain and surrender into the moment. Here is where the brain, mind, and body become one. The moment on the mountain becomes all there is. I step exactly where I should. This is the essence of flow. As soon as I think about stepping where I should, my foot misses, and pain follows.
HIGH ALTITUDE TRAINING	High altitude training refers to a type of athletic training that involves exercising or living at high altitudes (typically above 2,500 meters or 8,000 feet) to improve physical performance by increasing the body's ability to transport and use oxygen more efficiently.

HIP CARS	CAR is an acronym for Controlled Articular Rotations, which is a fancy way of saying, "moving the joint through its full range of motion." Hip CARs are performed by moving one's hips through their full range of motion. The purpose of this task is to improve hip mobility.
INTENSITY	Intensity has a few meanings in strength and conditioning. In classic strength training, intensity is a percentage of 100 and refers to the difficulty of the resistance compared to the most you can lift with that movement. For example, if my max squat is 100 pounds and I train with 70 pounds, then my intensity is 70% (70 pounds divided by 100 pounds). Intensity has other meanings. In CrossFit, coaches use the classic definition, as well as more subjective measures. Intensity can also refer to how hard an athlete is pushing in a workout. Without direct measuring with expensive and cumbersome equipment, estimating training intensity is completely subjective. If I completed a conditioning workout with burpees and pull-ups, I could assess my intensity for the workout based on how I "feel." Commonly, coaches utilize a 1–10 rating called Rate of Perceived Exertion, abbreviated RPE. Objective measures of output are more easily assessed with machine-based tasks like running, rowing, skiing, and biking. These tasks offer objective intensity tracking based on physical output. Output is often measured by tracking pace (miles per hour, kilometers per hour, or meters per minute), calories per hour, and most commonly in research settings, watts.
LACTATE	Lactate, also known as lactic acid, is a byproduct of anaerobic metabolism that accumulates in the muscles during high-intensity exercise. It is produced when the body breaks down glucose for energy in the absence of sufficient oxygen. Lactate is often used as a marker of exercise intensity. With regular training, the body can become more efficient at utilizing lactate as an energy source, leading to improved endurance and performance.
MALÖRT	Malört is a type of bitter liqueur that originated in Sweden and is traditionally made from wormwood and other herbs. It has a strong, pungent taste that is often described as bitter and herbal, with notes of citrus and anise. It is commonly consumed as a digestif or aperitif and is popular in the Chicago area as a regional specialty. To be honest, it's the worst tasting liquor in the world. If you are at a bar that serves Malört, if you buy shots for all your friends, the bartender may ask, "Do you hate your friends?"

METCON	A Metcon, in the CrossFit world, is shorthand for metabolic conditioning, which is a term used to describe a training strategy that relies on combining strength training, gymnastics, and cardiovascular training methods together into one intense and (usually) short training session. Metcons are a type of HIT (High Intensity Training) and HIIT (High Intensity Interval Training).
MUSCLE FIBER DISTRIBUTION	Muscle fibers can be categorized as Type I or Type II. Type I fibers are slow twitch, meaning they fire slowly, enabling resistance to fatigue, and are great for endurance tasks. Compared to Type I fibers, Type II fast twitch muscle fibers are significantly larger in diameter and are capable of faster firing rates. They fatigue more quickly than Type I fibers, but before they do, they produce a lot more force. They are the muscle fibers that support fast, explosive, and heavy tasks like weightlifting, carrying heavy things, sprinting, jumping, throwing, punching, and kicking. The fun stuff.
OVERTRAINING	Overtraining syndrome occurs when an athlete's training stressors outweigh their body's ability to recover. Over a few weeks to months, this imbalance can cause a plethora of unwanted outcomes, such as: • Underperformance • Staleness • Fatigue/low energy • Burnout • Injury • Reduction in desire to train • Fat gain • Muscle loss • Changes in bodyweight • Loss of appetite
PACK TEST	To enter rookie training, smokejumpers must complete a 110-lb. pack test on a flat 3-mile course in under 90 minutes for the USFS, and under 65 minutes for the BLM.
PEAKING	Peaking refers to a period in which an athlete is trained to achieve maximum performance potential for a specific competition or event. This involves a strategic approach to training that emphasizes optimal physical and mental conditioning and involves a tapering of training volume and intensity leading up to the event to allow for full recovery and optimal performance. Peaking is often used in sports that have a defined competitive season or schedule, such as track and field, swimming, and gymnastics, among others. Since smokejumpers also have a defined schedule, peaking is ideal for them, too.

PERFORMANCE AROUSAL THEORY	Performance Arousal Theory is sometimes referred to as The Inverted U Model of Arousal due to the shape of the curve when the theory is graphed. I like to call the shape an arch instead of an inverted U because an arch has two sides that uphold it, and the center piece on top, the keystone, keeps the arch from crumbling. The theory suggests that performance is optimized at an intermediate level of arousal (the keystone). Overarousal stimulates too much adrenaline and not enough motor and cognitive control. Underarousal fails to stimulate an appropriate response to the situation.
PLANTAR FASCIITIS	Plantar fasciitis is a painful inflammation of the thick band of tissue that runs across the bottom of the foot, connecting the heel bone to the toes.
PLYOMETRICS	Plyometrics, named "shock method" or "shock training," was first developed by sport scientist Yuri Verkhoshansky in Russia in 1959 and published in the Bulletin of the Central Research Institute of Physical Culture. The method initially prioritized the depth jump, which is a drop from the top of a box and either landing only (depth land), or dropping, landing, and then immediately jumping vertically for maximum height (depth jump). Today, there are seemingly endless variations of plyometric training tasks.
RHABDOM-YOLYSIS	Rhabdomyolysis is a serious medical condition characterized by the breakdown of muscle fibers, leading to the release of their contents into the bloodstream, which can cause damage to the kidneys and other organs.
RIG	A rig is a person that looks like a titanium brick with human features. Pure muscle. A physical specimen. Formidable. Infinitely capable. The root source of this word comes from outfitting a ship for sea, that is, making the ship as capable as possible to weather the storms it may encounter.
SMOKEJUMPER	Smokejumpers parachute out of planes to prevent forest fires from spreading. They are an elite branch of wildland firefighters who are called in, frequently first (along with helitack crews), and often for small forest fires that start from lightning strikes and other natural and sometimes unnatural means. They work in crews and jump out of nine different bases across the West Coast and the Pacific Northwest, namely California, Idaho, Montana, Oregon, Washington, and Alaska.

SUPER-COMPENSATION	Supercompensation is a process in which the body responds to training stress by overcompensating, leading to improved fitness and performance beyond the pretraining levels. During the recovery period following training, the body repairs and rebuilds tissues, and if given enough time and proper nutrition, it can achieve a state of supercompensation, when the muscles and other systems are stronger, faster, and more resilient than before. The goal of many training programs is to time the training and recovery periods to maximize the benefits of supercompensation.
TAPERING	A taper in sports preparation refers to a period of reduced training load, typically in the weeks leading up to an important competition, with the goal of optimizing an athlete's physical and psychological readiness for peak performance. The purpose of a taper is to balance the athlete's recovery and rest with their need to maintain or improve fitness and performance. During the taper period, the athlete gradually reduces training volume and intensity, allowing the body to recover from the accumulated fatigue of previous training, which allows the body to peak, maximally enhancing their performance potential.
TRAINING BLOCKS	In training design, many coaches break training blocks into microcycles, mesocycles, and macrocycles. Microcycles are the shortest, usually a week. Mesocycles are longer and consist of 3–8 microcycles lasting 1–2 months. Mesocycles are the largest and comprise several mesocycles, lasting 3–12 months. In classic periodization models, each microcycle within a mesocycle contains a specific amount of volume, and each block is different than the previous. The mesocycle structure I used for Heidi increased the volume each week for four weeks, and then the beginning of the next block served as a deload when the volume was decreased to allow for recovery.
TUMO BREATHING "WIM HOF"	Wim Hof breathing is a style of breath that upregulates sympathetic nervous system stimulation through hyperventilation. This specific style is similar to ancient Tummo breathing which dates back to texts from the eighth century, more than 1,200 years ago.

VOLUME	Volume refers to a specific amount of physical work. Units can be based on repetitions, distance (feet, meters, miles), duration, and total resistance. For bodyweight tasks like pull-ups or push-ups, volume is the total number of repetitions. For weightlifting, the volume is often calculated by multiplying the number of repetitions by the resistance. For example, if an athlete back squatted 100 pounds for 30 reps, the total volume would be 3,000 pounds (100 lbs. x 30 reps).
VOLUME TOLERANCE	Volume tolerance is an athlete's ability to recover from specific volumes of training stress. We can calculate training volume by multiplying the number of total repetitions completed by the resistance. Here are three simple examples of how to calculate for three different training stimuli: • 30 barbell back squats at 100 pounds = 30 x 100 = 3,000 pounds (back squat volume) • 3 days in one week with pull-ups, total reps = 250 (pull-up volume) • 120 miles of running completed in one month (month volume) You can track pounds lifted, miles run and hiked, repetitions completed, and training duration in minutes or hours. Once volume is calculated, you can compare that with your athlete's recovery data while undergoing that volume to decide how much to push them next time.
WAVE CYCLE	Wave cycles utilize progressive loading of training volume over a mesocycle. Imagine a month of training during which the first week is easy, the second week is a little tougher, the third tougher still, and the fourth is toughest. Four-week mesocycle complete! The next four-week mesocycle may contain a little more volume in each week, culminating in week 8 with the highest volume yet, higher than week 4s peak.
WEIRD WALKS	I learned these from Mike Erb. I first saw him instruct his athletes to perform these in a sand volleyball court in March once the rough Midwestern winter had died down. Walking up on the balls of the feet, walking on the heels, walking on the inner arches, and walking on the outer arches. Mike called these barefoot walks, but the athletes complained that they were weird, so I renamed them "weird walks."
WILDLAND FIREFIGHTING	Wildland firefighting consists of several different firefighting groups, including hand crews, engine crews, fuel crews, hotshots, helitack, wildland fire modules, and smokejumpers.

Printed in the USA
CPSIA information can be obtained
at www.ICGtesting.com
LVHW011619230624
783822LV00019B/37/J

STANISLAVSKY AND GENDER

Stanislavsky and Gender explores the intimate and complicated relationship between the enduring influence of Konstantin Stanislavsky and the evolving phenomenon of gender. This book provides new insights through historical research, unpublished and newly translated materials, and contemporary perspectives from diverse scholars and practitioners.

Readers will gain a nuanced understanding of how gender informs and intersects with the legacy of Konstantin Stanislavsky and its related traditions from historical, feminist, pedagogical, intersectional, and queer contexts. *Stanislavsky and Gender* combines historical and contemporary perspectives from scholars and practitioners from the UK, Ireland, the US, Australia, Russia, and Brazil. Their contributions cover theatre histories, her-stories, emotion, feminism, pedagogy, intersectionality, race, and queerness. Following each chapter, contributors are joined in conversation to discuss their writing in a broader context.

Part of the "Stanislavsky And…" series, *Stanislavsky and Gender* will be invaluable to scholars, teachers, students, and practitioners interested in integrating perspectives on gender into their research, teaching, and practice of Stanislavsky's legacy and associated traditions, and theatre history, acting, directing, actor training, and pedagogy more broadly.

Mark Shields (They/Them) is a queer nonbinary Postgraduate Researcher in Actor Training Pedagogy at the School of Performance and Cultural Industries, University of Leeds, UK. Mark is also a graduate of the Royal Central School of Speech and Drama, with an MA in actor training and coaching (2016) and of the University of Leeds (2011). Mark has also trained in teaching the Uta Hagen technique with HB Studio, New York, and holds Fellowship of the Higher Education Academy.

Stanislavsky And...

Series Editor: Paul Fryer

Stanislavsky And... is a ground-breaking new series of edited collected essays, each of which explores Stanislavsky's legacy in the context of issues of contemporary relevance and impact.

Drawing upon a unique series of webinars, symposia and study events presented as part of The S Word research project, each volume will focus upon a specific topic, utilising the expertise of a wide range of scholars and practitioners. A variety of written forms are supplemented by suggestions for studio work and exercises encouraging the widest possible practical exploration of the topic.

The series presents topics in a highly accessible form. It will appeal to students, teachers and practitioners at all levels, as well as those who wish to expand upon their knowledge of contemporary theatre practice and will positively encourage the development of new scholarship in the field.
Volumes currently available in the series are:

Stanislavsky and Race
Questioning the "System" in the 21st Century
Siiri Scott and Jay Paul Skelton

Stanislavsky and Intimacy
Joelle Ré Arp-Dunham

Stanislavsky and Gender
Mark Shields

For more information about this series, please visit: www.routledge.com/Stanislavsky-And/book-series/STAS